PUBLIC ENEMY #1: COVID-19

HOW A SINGLE VIRUS BROUGHT HUMANITY TO ITS KNEES.

JOSEPH W GRIECO

"When the people fear the government, there is tyranny; when the government fears the people, there is liberty."

Thomas Jefferson

HOW A SINGLE VIRUS BROUGHT HUMANITY TO ITS KNEES

Content Disclosure

Let it be known, by all who willingly choose to read the following script, that the content is biased. Need it also be mentioned that all the media coverage of COVID-19 that the World Health Organization, 'Big Pharma', Center for Disease Control, and Government coverage, are also extremely biased and not wholly based in fact. A truly unbiased work would only be feasible if produced in a literary vacuum, where facts are proven by reality and are delivered by a unanimous source of evidence that upholds over the courses of time. Bearing the preceding truths and the notions therewith, read on with your own rational mind and moral heart as your compass and measure. I urge you to contemplate the following opinions and stipulations without ignorance or defiance, whether you agree or not, if only for the duration of time it takes to read this text through. For it is considered an act of genius to be able to receive and contemplate the ideas and opinions of another party with whom disagreement is present, without ever changing one's own opinions and notions about a topic of moot interest. To act ignorant or to spray venom at another idea or party contrary to one's own, is an act of insecurity and stupidity. In the following piece, there is but one moot topic of elevated interest that is to be discussed. If not for the argument of validity, the piece will compare and contrast the declarations from both those who are in favor of the belief that *The Corona Virus Disease of 2019* is truly a deadly pandemic and that the vaccines that are being pressed and praised are but vehicles of hope and savior for all the people in the world, and those who are under the impression that the COVID-19 pandemic is an act of furtive population manipulation and control and that the various vaccines are a vehicle of pecuniary gain for elites and reproductive stinting for the common populace.

Note to the Reader!

Dear Reader,

I would first like to thank you for choosing to join me as we look at the growing chaos in the world, through a window of dichotomy. From the time most of us were very young, we have been exposed to a world and society full of people and things that do not agree. Primordial as it may be, the relationship between the consumed and the consumer, even provides evidence of nature's proclivity to disagree. It is fair for one to assume that the water buffalo acts in favor of its survival while the lion acts in favor of its demise. Be reminded, that even nature is full of a myriad of tiny disagreements. My own opinions surrounding the COVID-19 era, may or may not be in accord with your own. However, I did not write this book to continue a war between society and truth, people and government, law and heresy. With the purist motivation to pull the curtain of censorship and manipulation from unknowing eyes, I took up the onerous task of writing the words herein. The material has been carefully gathered from sources existing on either end of this argument of validation. It is meant to proffer those who are merely exposed to one side, a sift, of which to screen information freely and without the pollution from media and forced government hearsay. But you cannot convince a person who has perfect vision that they aren't blind, when they refuse to open their eyes, simply because some distant voice tells them to keep them closed. Human to human, I invite you to open your eyes. Learn from those whom you may disagree instead of lamenting over their position.

To the families of those who have fallen into the eternal sleep over the past year, I send my warm condolences. For those of us who are still living, I send you only positive vibes and high spirits. It is a depressing time for all humanity and like how any species is agitated when forced into captivity, we are frustrated to be barred by restrictions. Need I mention, time is life's trainer and its great revealer. May you strive for happiness and greatness in all the ways that you can, and may you embrace those whom you cherish and love the most. Moments make memories and may yours be, yet many filled with freedom and bliss.

Joseph W Grieco

Copyright 2020 by Joseph W Grieco

All rights reserved. This book may not be reproduced in whole or in part, stored in a retrieval system, or transmitted in any form or by any means electronic, mechanical, or other without written permission from the author, except by a reviewer, who may quote brief passages in a review.

This version was published via Amazon KDP

HOW A SINGLE VIRUS BROUGHT HUMANITY TO ITS KNEES

Content

The Beginnings of an End

•

Wuhan to President Trump

•

Europe Shuts Down

•

US and World Lockdown

•

Media Blizzard

•

A Sunny Day

•

Lockdown Two & Three

•

Florida: A Movement?

•

Vaccine Banter & Release

•

Political Storms & Side Effects

•

Freedom of Health & We the People

The Beginnings of an End

"COVID is a funhouse mirror that is amplifying issues that have existed forever. People are not dying from COVID. They are dying of racism, of economic inequality and it is not going to stop with COVID."

Shreya Kangovi, M.D., M.S.H.P., Professor at UPENN

No different than any other December in Wuhan, China, the sky wore a deep and smoggy gray mask. A blanket of fog was said to have accompanied an incessant light rain. It was the year 2019 and the rest of the world was busy existing as it had the year before. Like most of the modern superpowers in the world, The People's Republic of China does an excellent job of keeping its agendas in-house. With foggy-like mystery, the world gained reason to turn its attention to a laboratory in Hubei's capital. Popular stipulation of foul play began to accumulate after the outbreak of a new strand of SARS-CoV-2. Officials and eyewitnesses shared disturbing footage and evidence of unclean and illegal wet markets. Despite China's attempts to assure the rest of the world that it has been combatting the issue for a time, distrust and rumor spread rapidly. Scientist began to elude that the sudden spillover occurred because of human consumption of either the horseshoe bat of China or the endangered Pangolin, smuggled from South America. Experts have also discovered several cases of spillover from mink farms in several different countries including the United States and various members within the EU. Thus, the belief that the pandemic was caused by a spillover from animals to humans, remains at the top of expert opinions in the scientific community. However, there is no such evidence yet to suggest that this theory is indefinitely true. In blackness, it is only by light that facts will be seen. Political prejudice aside, the frigid foggy capital of Wuhan is indeed the site of the first known case of COVID-19. Whether this new strand of *CoV* was synthetically and intentionally developed in a lab in said location, is merely an allegation. It is also an allegation that holds such stringent political bias. For this reason, it is important to remember to focus one's attention on the light or the facts, and not the darkness that preludes assumptions and allegations. Wisdom follows those who remember that there is no truer guide to direction than the stars in all their fixed glory. Polaris points to north as facts point to the truth.

News about COVID-19 ebbed and flowed from the first breaking story about Wuhan until February 20, 2020, when a patient in a hospital in Lombardy, Italy had apparently been identified as having been infected by the virus. Only twenty-four hours later, more than thirty cases were identified.

In hindsight, how were doctors so quick to identify and test for this virus if proper tests were not even established until months down the line? Based on simply facts, science, and on what the W.H.O. and CDC have stated properly identifying the virus would not have been possible at this time. To question even further, how those reports could have been so quickly trusted when even current tests have proven to sometimes produce false results. (fda, 2021).

From the end of February, things began to heat up. Leaders were encouraging citizens to limit their travel and to avoid public gatherings whenever possible to do so. At this point, restrictions on travel were not a reality nor were the cancelling of all public gatherings such as concerts or cinemas. Despite the alleged case of COVID on the continent, the mere idea of being restricted from traveling remained taboo for most people around the world. On several occasions, my friends and I freely traveled throughout Italy and the EU without any issues or concerns. Not one time, was it required to wear a mask or to stay six feet apart. While in Madrid, I attended a Flamenco performance and later enjoyed a meal at a ritzy place off a main street downtown. This was still in February. By the time March had approached, I had already visited Stockholm, Sigtuna, Berlin, Tropea, and a few other places. Not once while either abroad or within Italy, did I witness a single case even vaguely resembling that of COVID-19. I had even mentioned to a friend, it seemed like the flu was taking a break this season. From one intelligent mind to another, does it seem vaguely improbable for a pandemic level virus to magically amass in such a short period of time without a trace? Would it make more sense that we all would have been hearing all about how severe the flu had been hitting everyone this year? There was more evidence to conclude that 2019 year was building up to be a good one compared to even 2018's flu season. Having lived in Italy, said to have been the world's worst hit nation, I had not seen any evidence that a pandemic was barking at the door. In actuality, life in Europe had been as cheery and delightful as ever. Some food for thought. But, like a bully tossing a dart into a child's balloon, the media and governments would quickly pop this buoyant aura.

On my return from a three-day getaway to the quiet isle of Wight, I entered the International Airport in Naples, Italy. To my astonishment, authorities in plastic face-shields and cloth masks, ushered us travelers into a que after holding an unfamiliar instrument up to our foreheads. Having just arrived from a beautiful and relaxing vacation, this took me by surprise. Before I had left the city of Naples, I had been casually following the latest stories surrounding the COVID-19 breakout in China. In keeping honest, I did not think very much of it. How could a stupid virus in one Chinese city possibly affect me here in Italy, let alone everyone in the entire world? Moments into being treated like cattle, I began to surge with fear. Maybe I had been too passive about Wuhan after all.

To the whole country's surprise, on March 9th, 2020, President Conte placed Italy into a national lockdown. Only those who were labeled essential, were permitted to commute to and from work but not without a written form notating a place of residence, destination, and duration of departure. During this first lockdown, even military members worked as little as two days per week. Grocery stores were policed by armed authorities known as the Carabiniere and ordered to strictly limit its occupancy during any given time. Streams of ques stretched out of the parking lot and down the street. Only weeks later, news of supply shortages hit the public. In some places, it was extremely difficult to find items such as hand sanitizer or toilet paper left in stock. Restaurants, shopping malls, bars, cinemas, cafes, and any place of business other than postal or grocery stores were forced to

HOW A SINGLE VIRUS BROUGHT HUMANITY TO ITS KNEES

shut down. If this was not already stressful enough, the Italian government began handing out penalties for leaving one's place of residence without a form. Depending on the day, these penalties could call for a person to pay hundreds of euro and even face time in prison. Media from around the world broadcasted nothing but frenetic hysteria and allegations. Even in its beginning, I often thought it would behoove of them to be sharing news of hope and positivity instead of hysteria and hopelessness. On week two, pick-up trucks equipped with giant speakers, began to patrol the neighborhood streets reminding people to remain indoors at all times and that disobeying would result in them facing severe penalties. Police check points began popping up everywhere. On two separate occasions, I was flagged to pool over by the infamous Italian lollipop that law enforcement uses to signal a vehicle to pull aside. An American, they often checked my form and NATO identification card and sent me on my way to either base or home. For my Italian neighbors, I felt a great sympathy. Every day, police vehicles pursued passing cars and forced them to pull aside. One night, police raced down an old man on his bike who was returning home and presented him with a penalty. I am not an Italian citizen but seeing this broke my heart. These free citizens were being treated like criminals. Less than a month earlier, I had been traversing to brilliant cities and embracing the various happy cultures across Europe. How could something this drastic have appeared and taken hold of society so suddenly? There had been no signs of a deadly virus having made landfall. It became very clear that we had entered the beginning of the end of life as we knew it.

For those who are not aware, humanity has faced famine since the dawn of time. Many of which, based on factual evidence, were far worse than the COVID-19 virus which at its climax, only reached a mortality rate of .01% on a world scale. Most recently, the Middle East Respiratory Virus, which is also caused by the coronavirus, is recorded to have had an estimated mortality rate of 35% (who.int, 2021). Strangely, the MERS-CoV had been reported in far less nations yet still proved to be more deadly than the present day COVID-19 virus. There was never a mass production or a worldwide urgent push for trial vaccinations during the

MERS-19 outbreak despite it proving to be more deadly than COVID-19. Unlike the current day COVID-19 pandemic, there were no worldwide government lockdowns, penalties for not wearing a mask, required forms to leave one's residence, restrictions and bans on travel, during the MERS-CoV outbreak. This information has been gathered from the same source that hoists the COVID-19 to the top of the list for the most horrible outbreaks in human history and it is not from myself or any other bias party. The International World Health Organization posts this information on its public website where anyone with internet access can visit and view just as I have. Facts do not lie…people lie.

Of all the times to scream and throw a tantrum, there is no better time then during a storm. There was not a single news station that was not talking about the COVID-19 pandemic and the varying measures governments around the world were placing on its people in an attempt to control the spread. Media pushed the government and the various health organizations atop a pedestal equivalent to that of a war hero or good Samaritan. Was this push merited? Perhaps there were and are government leaders and elite enterprises who have merely been trying to protect their people from the beginning. Could it also be possible, that by bloating these parties, media was distracting the common populace from the demasked agendas of these leaders? Who will notice the screams over the storm? Who can realize the crimes against humanity while there is an eruption at their doorstep? The intelligent mind leaves room for all rational possibility. It is basic if/then psychology. If one believes that it is possible that *A* is true, then one must also believe in the possibility that *B* could be true as well. In stepping outside of the house, you are able to notice the weeds in the garden. By stepping inside again, you notice the dirt you have tracked in and onto the carpet. There is always an opposite opinion than that of your own. The sooner you are able to acknowledge and accept this, the more intelligent your own opinion will then become.

While the torrential rains of COVID-19 dampened the worlds spirits and its strikes of fear, struck through the mass media, a political coocoo bird had snuck its way into the nest of the world's attention. President Donald J Trump, forty-

HOW A SINGLE VIRUS BROUGHT HUMANITY TO ITS KNEES

fifth president of the United States of America, was gathering a lot of negative attention from the world and the democratic party itself. It only made sense for a contending party to use a pandemic and world crisis to gain a political advantage. In the United States of America, politics are about as pure as the Yellow River in China. For those who are not aware of the ecological status of our friends in the east, the Yellow River is the most polluted river in the world. Instead of focusing on helping the people, political leaders in this country, too often focus on belittling the other. A US citizen myself, I am disheartened to see how far our once proud nation has stooped. It is a bipartisanship style government that has regressed into a rival war, where two parties under the same banner, bash one another leaving the population torn and vastly unsupported. This issue of grand division is not only a problem in the United States, but also an issue everywhere in the world. What most of the population fails to realize about division and prejudice, is that gender, race, religion, and orientation, are tadpoles whereas the economical prejudice is the frog. None of the tadpole issues matter if one is a member of the elite class. If one is a frog that has grown to hop right on out of the pond of stirred water. Locked inside with nothing to do, the world was one giant waiting ear eager to be filled with more information.

Wuhan to President Trump

"Falsehood flies, and truth comes limping after it, so that when men come to be undeceived, it is too late; the jest is over, and the tale hath had its effect: like a man, who hath thought of a good repartee when the discourse is changed, or the company parted; or like a physician, who hath found out an infallible medicine, after the patient is dead."

Jonathan Swift, Irish Satirist & Political Pamphleteer

Look at a house and admire its many windows and evaluate its few entrances. Both windows and doors can be either opened or closed. It is truthful to state that any sane owner would wish to keep both windows and doors closed from unwanted visitors such as thieves or pests. If there is a wife or a daughter undressing upstairs, it would be natural she would wish to be concealed by curtains or blinds, otherwise, uninvited eyes may find themselves peeping inside. Treat your mind like you would treat your home. For the ears are like doors and the eyes like windows. It is true, that the mouth can cause a person great harm or benefit, but the information that is received is oftentimes what manipulates and determines what filth or magic may come out of the mouth. Take care when you are deciding what types of information to receive through hearing or seeing. Modernity and technology have made the dissemination of information easier than ever before. Author of *The American Paradox: Spiritual Hunger in an Age of Plenty,* well known psychologist David Myers, warns that materialism and radical individualism have gravely distorted people's ability to discern what information is healthy and what information is not. It eludes me to conject that maybe Mr. Myers was on to something and that his writings and psychology prove truer today than even at the time when he wrote this book. Are we too quick to believe everything that we hear from news stations or world leaders? Do we even stop and consider the things that are being broadcasted? Are our political decisions influenced or even dependent upon a positive reaction on a social media platform?

HOW A SINGLE VIRUS BROUGHT HUMANITY TO ITS KNEES

It is most prudent to learn the properties of a plant before consuming it because of course, it could prove to be poisonous. Why then do so many of us take what we hear or see as truth the very instant that we hear or see it? Should we not treat the information that we receive with the same careful observation? For what, if what you heard on social media, proves to have been a lie and for a time, you lost friendships over defending a point which was never your own to begin with and a point that you never digested and observed before swallowing into your belief system? Even worse, what if you had taken to arms for a cause that you later learned was furtive genocide? Do not be fooled; not everyone in Hitlers evil ranks knew what was afoot. I am not urging you to take a particular side in the argument over the validity of COVID-19 or the politics of the world. I am however, encouraging you to be a student of yourself; one who stops to review and interpret the information that he or she receives before bringing an outside agenda or opinion into your own nest. The best way a student can excel at a test is by reviewing the facts and studying the material. Next time you are scrolling through social media or listening to the news, mentally masticate or chew, the information, before you swallow it. For example, if you are a citizen in Turkey and a reporter is speaking about chaos in America, before believing that people have went crazy across the Atlantic, research the current status of America or actually speak to an American. When we measure what we hear or see against the facts, we will know where the truth abides. Think of this process as sifting for gold, where the shaking of the pan is your fact checking and the gold that remains are the truths. Protect your mind from poisonous media and faulty information just as you would protect your body from a poisonous plant.

Evil is a snake. Evil can take whatever side it pleases and it will always take the side of the party who will cause the most harm. It thrives on an evergreen process of disguise and ecdysis. One such skin the snake of evil has worn during the pandemic, is that of United States politics and racism against people of darker skin pigment or of Chinese origins. No matter where I traveled to or what I did to avoid it, media ridiculing President Trump always sprang up. No matter what civil issue arose within the country, media blamed one person and one house. When

George Floyd was wrongfully shot and killed, media somehow extended blame to President Trump and all republicans somehow became racists and white. Crimes against a particular race or ethnicity have been around since the days of the Pharaoh. To blame a single man and one who was not present, no matter his position, is uproarious. Officer Chauvin is guilty of committing this racist act and all the officers who later committed the other hate crimes, are the culprits. But to label an entire race as being racist, an entire political party of consisting of only one race or singling out a man who was not even present, as being equally guilty, is an act of grand evil itself. Not only does one create a greater division between people whose particular difference being evaluated, is over simply skin pigment, one takes some of the weight off of the backs of those who actually pulled the trigger and have actually proven to be racist. Black or white, evaluate the facts before swallowing the pill media or peers place into your hands. Racism is the enemy, not the President of the United States because he happens to be white or not all white people because they are assumed to be racist by mass media. There are racist people who belong to all races because racism is a problem of the heart and not of the skin. A president is a good president, or a bad president based upon his or her ability to justly rule a nation. Focus on the facts and the problems will be easier to cut down. You would never bring a plastic knife to a lumber cutting party. It makes a lot more sense that the egotism in the American political system created a jaded agenda for media to stir unrest amongst the people in order to then use such unrest as a tool of blame against President Trump and the Republican party. Instead, what if Americans realized the facts, that there are good and bad people of both races and that when cut, we all bleed red, and when it comes to evil, it is an individual's morality that will determine an individual's actions. Racism is merely a blanket of laziness and ignorance to reality and truth. To an American who is living abroad, it is obvious to me that this was part of a political game of distraction. There has always been a snake of evil racism slithering its way through American society. Earth to America and the world: it was not a problem that was caused by President Trump and historical facts will prove that truth and nothing less. In stating any of the preceding examples, I am not

HOW A SINGLE VIRUS BROUGHT HUMANITY TO ITS KNEES

attempting to support President Trump, or the Republican Party nor am I attempting to demean the Democratic Party and its members. I am merely using facts to illuminate false information and media-manipulation. Facts do not lie…people lie. The Great Martin Luther King said it best,

"We must live together as brothers or perish together as fools."

According to NBC News, Anti-Asian hate crimes increased by 150% in 2020. There have been mass shootings in schools, at concerts, in theatres, against religious groups, and homosexuals. Stop swallowing the pills of media. Racist and prejudice crime is an issue that effects far more than just two races. Evil is a snake of many different skins. One day it may wear the color white, the next black, and the following day, the colors of the Chinese or LGBTQ flags. Process information before acting on what you hear or see and weigh the validity of its source by holding it up to what is known fact. Could China have developed a strand of the Coronavirus in a lab in Wuhan to cause disruption in the world? It is possible. But it is also equally as possible the pandemic was caused by experiments within a lab in the United States. For anyone to be expressing prejudice against Asians or China itself for the COVID-19 pandemic, is deplorable and inaccurate. When the origins of the virus are excavated and proven by concrete fact, it will be fair to place blame and aim anger. To further my point on the nature of democratic media, ridiculing President Trump for calling the COVID-19 virus the "Chinese Virus", is yet another attempt to sway the election. It took Donald Trump becoming President for the world to suddenly find it offensive for someone to refer to a virus by its country or nation of origin? Last I checked, there are no Spaniards insulted by the name *Spanish Flu* or Muslims who are offended by the *Middle East Respiratory Syndrome-related coronavirus* label. So, ask yourself why it would benefit American politics or an elite party's agenda, to suddenly create a problem where one never existed in the history of world health? The objective is not to convince you to believe something other than what you may believe in. It is entirely to convince you to consider and to contemplate the notions you believe about the ongoing situation. By asking yourself the questions

I have written and those akin, you will better understand why you may have taken a particular stance. Personally, I am not a fan of being locked inside my house like an animal in a zoo nor am I in favor of being told to wear a mask for extended periods of time when facts reveal its ineffectiveness at preventing a virus and its harmful effects to my overall health. Are you not at least a little curious about discovering whether all that you are being told is true or false when held against facts? What if in two years, you learn that COVID-19 and all the civil storms that followed, were in fact part of a greater and more sinister plan? Have you measured the possibility that that evil snake has taken COVID-19 as its very skin to gain power over the masses? How angry would you be if you learned that you had spent the greater part of the last year locked down and faceless all for smokescreen and false information used to manipulate and gain control? How much angrier would you be if you had lost your business as a result or failed to experience college because the restrictions forced you to learn from behind a screen? None of the questions I am leaving you to consider may come true. But, if there is a chance that they will prove to be false, there is an equal chance that they will prove to be true. Facts do not lie…people do.

HOW A SINGLE VIRUS BROUGHT HUMANITY TO ITS KNEES

Europe Shuts Down

"Power is tearing human minds to pieces and putting them together again in new shapes of your own choosing."

George Orwell, 1984

By the fifteenth of March, leaders in the European Union had placed a universal travel ban on all citizens within the Schengen zone. President Trump responded by banning all non-essential travel from the European Union to the United States. Before March was over, Europe was locked down and ordered to stay at home. Italy maintained its lead position as the worst effected nation in the world with an average of nearly six-hundred recorded cases per seven-day period. This figure would later be brought into question, when evidence revealed that hospitals were being bribed to skew numbers by recording every death as COVID-19. By doing so, a hospital, region, and ultimately, a nation, would receive more funding. Nothing like the promise of more money to motivate lying and manipulation. Keep in mind, that none of these facts of manipulation were discovered until much later. While media continued to report rising numbers of deaths and cases, people were bespelled into a hypnosis of fear. What better way exists than fear, to control a population to shut up and comply? Unbeknownst to the entire population, their civil rights were being stripped from them by an unjust ruling to implement Martial Law and Draconian rule. In ancient Greece, an official by the name of Draco issued extremely strict and unfair laws on his people. It is for this reason that we now use the word *Draconian* to describe rules and restrictions that are repressive, unruly, and harsh. While I was visiting the charming country of

PUBLIC ENEMY #1: COVID-19

Singapore, I was briefed about the country's draconian law that states that a person who is caught chewing gum can be sentenced to up to two years in prison and fined for upwards of one hundred thousand Singapore Dollars. For the entirety of my stay, I opted for mints and avoided foods containing garlic. As ludicrous as the severity may seem to the westerner, Singaporean leaders justify the law by reminding citizens and travelers of its previous problem with vandals leaving spent gum in mailboxes, keyholes, and in places meant to disrupt public services. When viewed in light of these facts, it is hard to argue with this measure.

However, when it comes to the issuing of draconian laws during the ongoing pandemic, I find no such facts to support the issuance of such harsh and repressive measures. Prohibiting people from chewing gum does not negatively affect a person's health or wellbeing nor does it corrode an economy or cause the working class to suffer. Prohibiting people from living their lives by ordering them to stay home and to close business, greatly and negatively affects their health and wellbeing. Never in the history of the world, has human travel been reduced as severely as it has this past year and a couple of months. The draconian bans on movements have caused the tourism and travel industry to lose more than seven hundred and fifty billion dollars. With a death rate of a skyrocketing .01%, it only seems necessary to ground planes and run millions of businesses into the ground, wouldn't you agree? I ask the preceding rhetorical question sarcastically. This deficit has only increased since the new year. According to the CDC itself, mental health issues and depression have risen to unprecedented levels since the lockdowns were first implemented. Statistics from the government source show that the same polls on mental health issues taken from a year prior to COVID-19, have increased by almost 50%. Millions of workers have reported that they have lost their job as a result of the COVID-19 lockdowns and stars-worth of businesses were forced to close permanently or until governments developed sufficient plans to provide financial aid. It is more heart wrenching when one considers the economic effect on a global scale. Will these smaller governing bodies even be able to recover or to provide its business owners relief? Many have still failed to offer such aid after more than a year. In Naples, Italy there are numerous families who have maintained businesses based on tourism and daily attendance for centuries. Being forced to close shop not only severs the family's only means of income, but it also decimates its morale and pride. Many countries like the United States and Italy, have provided its citizens with stimulus checks hoping to aid their financially crippled populations. A step in a positive direction but one that would have never been necessary if leaders had acted based on fact instead of only fear or lust for power and control.

History is full of salmon, pioneers, people who go against the current. Too many of humanity's great discoveries were first neglected and ridiculed by society and its leaders. Take Galileo, Copernicus, Semmelweis, Pasteur, and Pythagoras for example. Both Galileo and Copernicus were persecuted for their beliefs in heliocentrism, Semmelweis was disregarded for his theories on antiseptics, Pasteur proved the existence of bacteria, yet it took the field of medicine years to finally recognize his masterwork, and Pythagoras was the first person in history to challenge the idea that the world was flat, but his idea was quickly dismissed for centuries. What all of these fascinating and pivotal discoveries have in common, is that they were originally widely unaccepted and often ridiculed, only to later be accepted and proven to be true. During the COVID-19 pandemic, anyone who challenges the information produced by governments, elites, CDC, W.H.O., or even social media platforms, is immediately dismissed and labeled as either a Trump rightest, a racist, or a conspiracy theorist. An educated and extremely well-read mind, I find this name-calling and mislabeling to be blatantly childish and utterly defensive. What are these entities hiding that they feel the need to belittle any idea that opposes or even questions their own? It is considered genius to be able to listen and receive another's ideas or arguments without demeaning them or changing one's own ideas or stance. By definition, all of these agencies have been acting without genius and from under a cloak of sketchiness. How is it, that every time a person posts any information about COVID-19, they are issued a message from the CDC or W.H.O. informing viewers that the post had been reviewed by their "fact-checkers" and to click to see all true material? Why would these parties care about a person posting about an opinion that opposes the lockdowns or highlights evidence of how numbers have been manipulated since the beginning? The only reason anyone would care about the sun rising on their plans, is if they know that they are guilty and they are trying to conceal secrets and cover up lies.

The following are examples of such messages one will receive on social media after posting anything remotely contesting the validity of COVID-19, vaccines, and the draconian measures surrounding it.

False Information: Checked by Independent Fact Checkers

COVID-19 vaccine development was accelerated without impacting public safety.

Vaccines are thoroughly tested for safety before they are approved.

Vaccine side effects are usually mild.

Vaccine trials involve a diverse range of volunteers.

COVID-19 vaccine trials are following safety and ethical standards.

On a few occasions, a post will be deleted, or the content will be blurred behind a message stating that the information that was being presented was fact checked by the organizations third-party, whomever that may be. Most of the above scripts were sourced from the World Health Organizations on Instagram and are oriented around the vaccines because of the current controversy that surrounds the safety of said trial vaccines. The vaccines will be addressed in more detail in a later chapter, but it is necessary to mention that the validity behind most of the above statements of standard by social media, can be called into question by simply visiting separate pages within the WHO's webpage and viewing procedures and methods posted therein, that contradict each point that is being broadcasted as the standard of truth. What I am trying to convey now, is that there is an ongoing censorship of all information about COVID-19. A person should not have to go through government censorship to view or show evidence of one such W.H.O. or CDC report displaying fallacious information about the pandemic. In the United States of America, it is written in the Constitution that its citizens possess the freedom of press and speech. The exampled actions of censorship, directly abuse American citizens of this Constitutional right. These basic rights can be found to be true for many other nations as well. If you have read this far, you have probably gathered that I am an advocate for the truth and it is my belief, that the COVID-19 pandemic has many weeds in the garden. My ultimate goal is for the governing parties to validate this censoring and to bring to your attention, that it is afoot and that these actions are not constitutional. A weed is a wild plant growing where it is not wanted and in competition with cultivated plants (Oxford, 2021). When there are weeds in the garden, the only thing to do in order to protect the flowers, is to first distinguish the flowers from the weeds, and then get to digging and yank the weeds out by the roots!

Like the litany of pioneers, I mentioned in the previous paragraph, Sweden had decided to swim against stream and came out far better than those who did not. Epidemiologist, Anders Tegnell, lead the Scandinavian country's COVID-19 response plan. In spite of the world's ridiculing, Sweden has maintained some of the lowest numbers of verified cases and was able to maintain its economic health and quality of life. Swedish experts also share that almost all of the deaths were elderly ranging from seventy years of age or older. People were able to meet for a café or to enjoy a bike ride on a sunny day unlike any other European country and most of the world. Did Sweden make the right call? Or was ordering almost four billion people to stay home the right decision? The statistical evidence certainly proves Sweden made the better call.

In Italy, the first lockdown felt like living in the movie *Groundhog Day*. Many relationships were placed under an unprecedented amount of stress. For those who live alone, depression often hit harder and faster. It was not until early May that lockdown restrictions were eased in Italy. Being the country with the strictest and longest lockdown, the process of lifting bans occurred slowly. At first, citizens were only permitted to commute within one's own region. At the next step, we were able to travel throughout Italy but could not leave the country unless it was proven to be for essential travel. By late summer, a list of open countries was presented that allowed people to travel to and from these places without restriction. This mid-summer freedom seemed to be an attempt for the government to regain some of the economic losses it had incurred from a loss of tourism. The end of the summer also happens to mark the start of the infamous holiday known as Ferragosto across Italy. It was peculiar when announcements were made about predictions that a "second-wave" would hit the nation and Europe conveniently at the close of the busy tourist season and acclaimed holiday. Did the country only open its borders and end its lockdown to let out some pressure? The truth is destined to come out sooner than later, but the breather was much appreciated. However, it was short-lived. Italy and most of Europe closed the cage again in early October and November. As if by a stroke of magic, the number of cases began to rise over the exact period of time officials had warned that they would over the summer. What was different about the first lockdown? In the beginning, the population was led to believe it was being shackled to ensure to the safety of the weak of elderly. Once people realized this was not an appropriate or effective response, they began to rush the streets in rebellion. To gain back control, the W.H.O., government, media, and CDC, changed the story and began informing the population that the virus was now affecting people of all ages and that it was often "asymptomatic." An eighty-year-old man who was terminally ill with cancer is counted in the COVID-19 death tolls as well as almost every otherwise normal passing, of an elderly or sick citizen. Europe consists of countries with populations where the elderly outnumbers the youth. In many of these countries, illnesses such as the common flu, pneumonia, and cancer have plagued these nations for decades. If one quickly reviews the numbers showing the total number of cases and deaths for any of these illnesses, one will be shocked to see that these numbers have mysteriously plummeted. It is like the W.H.O. had discovered a cure for cancer! However, before you begin leaping for joy, compare these statistics with those of years leading up to COVID-19 outbreak. It is encouraged that you visit scholarly medical journals for your research and fact checks. Though, most of these discoveries can be made from viewing information right on the W.H.O. and CDC websites. A recent news headline in America reads: *CDC Numbers reveal hospitals counted over 130K deaths from Pneumonia, Influenza, Heart Attack, and Cancer, as COVID-19.* I am not a professional researcher, I am not a college professor, and I am not a member of the medical community. The facts and information I have gathered and gleaned about all the disinformation we have been given from the beginning can be searched and found by the least scholarly of us common people. What makes the difference between the easily manipulated person and the person who is sound in judgement, is rather simple. A person who has a sound judgement asks questions about the information that they hear or see, and they visit the facts before swallowing it up as truth.

Locking people into their homes for over three months is not ethical and it has caused far greater harm than it has benefit. The lockdowns have not managed to accomplish anything in Europe because according to the media's replication of the number of cases throughout, they continued to rise whether people were locked in-house or freely moving around. It begs one to question, why did they do it and why are they continuing to do it? It is a civil rights and ethical issue at large. Physician and Attorney Dr. Simone Gold, debunks the hysteria produced by mass media, government, W.H.O., and the CDC. In a speech conducted on April 8, 2021, she recounts actual statistics:

"I can assure you that I have thought about this issue of induvial liberty versus group safety a great deal. Under no circumstances, would SARS-CoV-2 (COVID-19) meet the threshold of abridging individual sovereignty. Let me remind everybody of the numbers of lethality and non-lethality of SARS-CoV-2 (COVID-19). If you are under twenty and you catch SARS-CoV-2, your chances of survival with no treatment at all is 99.997%. If you are between twenty and fifty and you contract SARS-CoV-2 (COVID-19) with no treatment at all, your chance of survival is 99.98%. If you are between fifty and seventy and you contract SARS-CoV-2 with no treatment at all, your chances of survival are 99.5%."

If you are like a majority of the world, you rely on media and governments to provide you with all the information that you need to remain updated and safe. It is also true, that if you rely solely on these sources, like too much of our world population, you trust these sources and therefore, rarely fact check whatever they inform you of. In an attempt to help people and to ensure they are truly safe and treated fairly, I strongly urge you to fact check them all. These real statistics are from the mouth of a professional with nothing to gain and everything to lose by pulling the mask off of this mass hysteria. Dr. Gold was fired for advocating the use of hydroxychloroquine to combat COVID-19. This proven effective treatment was once readily available anywhere in the world but was quickly removed from shelves in the United States and several other countries around the globe. This act alone is shameful and disturbing to say the least. If you are truly concerned about the safety and wellbeing of your people, you would readily provide any and all treatments that have proven to be effective. Instead, the W.H.O. and CDC recalled this panacea for COVID-19 and prescribed people to experimental vaccines. When you consider both sides of the argument, do the actions of the W.H.O. not seem at least slightly suspicious? There is only one reason an acclaimed, highly intelligent, and successful, doctor would jeopardize her role in medicine and that reason is to share a truth that is being hidden or blurred before the population's very eyes. Dr. Gold was one of the good doctors who sought to provide people with the truth that would best serve them. Did not Pasteur and Semmelweis experience similar contest when they produced their own evidence? The governing medical body of their times was behind them. They were clouded by their own pride and therefore missed years of preventing sickness and death and as a result, many died that otherwise would have been cured by the discoveries of these two individuals. It was only after time revealed the validity of their research that the governing medical party accepted and embraced them. Is it not also probable that the medical professionals that are being silenced, ridiculed, fired, and imprisoned, for speaking out about simple proven remedies for COVID-19, sharing true statistics, or warning against the dissemination of experimental vaccines, are truly sharing the truths? Is it possible that media has been kicking sand in the aridity of the situation, to intentionally hide a completely separate agenda? All I ask is that you consider the following question: How does it make you feel after learning that one of the busiest continents in the world was shut down for a virus that has nearly a one-hundred percent recovery rate for people of ages ranging from zero to seventy? U.S. Senator and Diplomat, Daniel Patrick Moynihan says,

"everyone is entitled to his own opinion, but not his own facts."

Let it be known fact, that in most of the countries in Europe, the government can legally enforce lockdowns and business restrictions. Government leaders have acted within legal bounds when issuing the COVID-19 lockdowns. However, the legal aspect of the lockdowns is not what the world is questioning. What the world is questioning and has a right to know, is, were they really merited and even necessary. Much of the information and facts gathered from experts in medical and scientific communities, would prove that they were in fact not. During the Spanish Flu, which had a much higher mortality rate than COVID-19 by a longshot, governments did not choose to utilize these legal but very extreme measures. It is also worth mentioning that laws are not always in the populations best interest. For example, in the past, it was also once legal for a government to seize members for royal use at any point. Due to major civil rights issues and cases of inhumanity, these laws have been banned in all the free world. It took millennia for these legal changes and civil rights protections to be instated. It is only plausible to state, that the same possibility could later prove to be true about these lockdowns and restrictions. As the discussion moves to the continent across the ocean and around the world, take a moment to dissect all that you have believed to be true about COVID-19 before reading this book or visiting the various professional sources available for fact checking. If there is one thing the European community can agree on, it is that we all want things to go back to the way that they were and to the way that they should be. There is no such thing as a *new normal*.

US and World Lockdown

"The first duty of a man is to think for himself."

Jose Marti, Cuban National Hero

With the media, there is always a motivation to hyperbolize and exaggerate. Regardless of whether a certain story or headline is fact or fallacy, the world's media will never fail to make it sound either worse or better than it actually is. From the dawn of time, human beings have been obsessed with either telling a story or listening to a story. As social beings, we have also always possessed a desire to be aware and informed. If there was a large predator wiping out a nearby village, it is beneficial for the neighboring village to become aware of the threat in order to properly prepare. When a grandfather sits his grandchild on his lap, he will often share stories of life and lessons. It is natural for humans to communicate. What is also natural, is for humans to lie for gain. Mass media has taken up this role and continues to twist and derange the truth in hopes of acquiring more viewers and in turn, reap more profits. In light of the COVID-19 pandemic, media has been handed all the materials needed to put on the performance of the century. It knows that most people in the world, simply receive and believe the information that they produce and disseminate. Since the start of the COVID-19 pandemic, the media has striven to instill fear into every household. Instead of caring about validity, they took reports from both publicly known and unknown sources and shared them as facts. These blatant violations of the truth have become evident as time went on. Reports have been made which counter previously promoted statistics such as those regarding the number of deaths and cases of COVID-19, once the disproving evidence had been disclosed. In other words, *they covered their asses*. While Europe was locked down, the United States was still deciding on whether it would follow suit and lockdown as well. Instead of providing real statistics, media in the United States portrayed

HOW A SINGLE VIRUS BROUGHT HUMANITY TO ITS KNEES

blatantly false stories of the COVID-19 situation in Italy. Some of the reports I have seen or been shown by friends and family who were living in the United States consisted of things such as military vehicles being needed to transport corpses and mass graves being constructed to accommodate all the deaths from COVID-19. These stories are the farthest thing from being true. I was living in Italy during this time and working for NATO and can promise the populace that such stories are bullshit. Another example of a false story produced by world media is about how President Trump was to blame for the thousands of deaths that would eventually be reported in the United States. Due to the discovery of recent evidence, the CDC, W.H.O., and mass media, have been nothing short of deceitful when sharing these statistics with US citizens and the world. A vast majority of the deaths recorded as COVID-19 being the cause, were in fact patients who died for a myriad of different reasons such as pneumonia, heart disease, influenza, and even natural causes. In the United States, including politics into a major health crisis was a bold and asinine move. In response to the pressure brought on by these stories, the President granted states the right to issue lockdowns which began on different dates starting from the end of March and into early April of 2020. This is not an attempt to support President Trump, but I believe he said it perfectly as he addressed the population about a report created to blame him for not initiating a lockdown at an earlier date:

"It was a political hit job."

The said reports were created by university students at Columbia and John Hopkins but to-date, they are vastly inaccurate as they came to their estimations by using numbers and statistics from W.H.O. and CDC that were later proven exaggerated and vastly inflated. Unlike in Europe, the lockdown situation in North America proved to be a political skirmish rather than a serious health concern. Mass media and political leaders stirred riots and authorities failed to enforce its own measures against the rioters who were clearly in violation of these COVID-19 measures. Certain states such as Florida, would emerge as defiant and outrageous according to world media and W.H.O., for choosing to remain open and in taking an approach similar to that of Sweden. Florida residents frequented beaches, enjoyed restaurants, socialized like human beings, and never had an explosion of cases or deaths as media and W.H.O. had forewarned. As time progressed and more and more reports about the government, CDC, and W.H.O., providing false and misleading numbers began to emerge, other states followed suit and decided to lift its lockdown measures. One of the leading faces of the battle against the COVID-19 pandemic is Dr. Fauci, Director of U.S. National Institute of Allergy and Infectious Diseases and chief medical advisor to the President. In a report written by Senator Marco Rubio, evidence emerged showing that Dr. Fauci had admitted he had selectively lied to the American public during an interview about the COVID-19 pandemic and what the country needed to do for its recovery. When the representative who is in charge of a nation's medical response admits that he has lied and evidence is produced to further validate this claim, any intelligent person would feel pressed to check the facts. In a world where there is so much deceit in media, communication of information has become about as trustworthy as it had been before the invention of the photograph or the recorder. In those days, a paper could produce a story in one city about another without ever having visited or experienced it for themselves. The gap between fact and fiction was great with too little technology and it is greater still with too much of it. Facts do not lie…people lie.

In many countries in Europe, the first lockdowns lasted longer than three months. In other places like the United States, it barely lasted a month. People will begin to question a story and to demand evidence to support claims especially after being saturated in induced hysteria. Government officials in a few states such as California and New York, upheld a stringent lockdown order. New York state governor, Andrew Cuomo has also been found guilty of withholding information from the public about COVID-19. It is becoming more and more clear that many of the faces at the front of this COVID-19 regime, are less than trustworthy. The State News declares,

"Cuomo's nursing home fiasco shows the ethical perils of policymaking."

HOW A SINGLE VIRUS BROUGHT HUMANITY TO ITS KNEES

On the other side of the country, California state governor, Gavin Newsom, faced a giant lawsuit for providing false statistics about COVID-19 being linked to fitness centers. The California Fitness Alliance had filed a lawsuit at the Supreme Court level arguing against the COVID-19 restrictions in place across the state and are proving to be victorious. There is no greater evidence of idiocy than an official fighting to prevent exercise. Unfortunately, measures that demote good health and exercise continue to remain in effect across the world. Here in southern Italy's Campania region, citizens were not permitted to even exercise outside. It is medically proven that a good exercise routine is essential to building a strong immune system. Nowhere in science, is it proven that taking a walk through the park is a dangerous thing to do during flu season. It seems rather contradictory for a leader to prevent a person from exercising in an attempt to prevent the spread of a virus that only has a potency against weakened immune systems. As a fitness nutrition specialist and elite trainer, myself, it is infuriating to be hindered in such an unjustifiably stupid manner. Kris Mulkey, Chief Marketing Officer of In-Shape Health Clubs, happily exclaims,

"We know that the data shows that we are not super-spreaders of COVID, and the data also shows how important fitness is for your mental and physical health. So, we are going to continue to fight so that people have more access. Outdoor fitness is great, but we don't have it everywhere and we want to be able to open up indoors."

As the lockdown was coming to a close in most states in the US, Senate passed the CARES Act which provided $2 trillion to help the country recover and further combat the pandemic. Receiving this borrowed money, most of the country stopped questioning and complaining. Much of the publicity was focused on blundering President Trump and promoting agendas of the Democratic Party. From an outside perspective, the United States political parties were heavily using the pandemic as a political tool to wield either against an opposing party or in favor of its own. Several other issues of civil unrest coincidentally arose over the course of the last year. Only incidences where *white Trump supporters* had committed heinous crimes against African Americans were circulated by mass media. Over the same period of time, an African American man shot and killed a white father and his daughter at point blank range in Georgetown County, South Carolina. There was never worldwide coverage or publicity of this equally heinous hate crime. As previously stated, racism is afoot amidst people of all races. In America and much of the western world however, it is portrayed as being strictly an issue of white on black racism. This demeans the seriousness of hate crimes and racism itself and further creates more hate between these two races. Mass media has proven time and time again that it will gladly stir the pot at any expense so long as it is guaranteed a profit. The media's failure to display the reality that racism is a major problem in the world amongst both people of light and dark skin pigment, is a great injustice. In the case of America, it is rather obvious that the media had started stirring this pot to create more hate against Donald Trump. As a result, there is more racism amongst the American people than there already was. All of these political and civil issues were being blended in with the rising tides of COVID-19 hysteria. This is simply another example of how deceitful and untrue mass media can be and proves its clever propensity to further or worsen the very issues it leads viewers to believe it wants to resolve. Check the facts before you go believing everything that you hear on media. If you are an African American: has every white person that you know, proven to be a racist backwards Trump supporter? If you are a Caucasian: has every black person that you know proven to be a democratic derelict? If you are being honest with yourself, the answer to both of those questions should be a resounding "*NO*". Do not be ignorant and naïve enough to believe that racism is one-sided. Further, do not be ignorant and naïve enough to believe that the timing of all these events has been merely coincidental.

To conclude the discussion about the lockdowns throughout the world, there is evidence eluding that they had little to no drastic effect on the number of cases or deaths. Take into consideration, there are no known true and factual statistics at this point due to proven exaggeration, scientifically unsound testing, and improper recording. However, slight variations in the number of reported cases can be evidenced via the many government and medical sites, which typically depict an increase during those periods where cases of influenza are regularly and historically higher. There is no proven correlation between the draconian measures and a drop in known cases or deaths. Intriguing evidence to suggest it has been more harmful than beneficial and therefore, pointless, can be deduced by the fact there has been three to four different attempts to issue said extreme measures. If a lockdown was as effective as mass media, government, and the W.H.O. encourage the population to believe, it would be hard to disagree that there would have been no necessity for the issuance of two to three more lockdowns of the same nature. Think for yourself. The power of the human mind does not derive from its ability to mime the thinking of other minds or to emulate the actions of other bodies. True mental strength and intelligence is in one's own ability to measure outside receptions by one's own thinking, values, principles, and factual observation. Without such an ability, what more does the mind become than a robotic recorder; what more does the body become than a slave to someone else's propaganda.

Media Blizzard

"When they give you lined paper, write the other way."

Ray Bradbury, Fahrenheit 451

When viewing the current unrest in the world, one must be careful to evaluate the education system of a nation. How are a nation's youth being taught? Are lectures about history being taught from the perspective of both sides of the battlefield or are teachers simply indoctrinating? Associate Editor of *Education Week*, Stephen Sawchuk, puts it this way,

"It's easy to lose sight of the connection between what students learn in history and the civic ideals and values those topics communicate, especially since they tend to be treated as different disciplines in K-12 education."

In many school systems around the world, teachers and education communities are peppering lessons with personal bias. As an instructor, one is held to a higher standard when it comes to avoiding teaching with bias or intention to dissuade one belief over the other. There is a serious issue of censorship and politically selective curricula in many schools around the world and particularly in the United States. Forcing propaganda and belief systems that support only the views of the democratic party onto the public youth is an outrageous example of indoctrination that is happening throughout the country since the election. Even people who have graduated on from the school system are feeling the radiation of such brainwashing. For example, all workplaces were forced to conduct trainings about equality in the workplace. On the surface, this is always an exemplar training to conduct in any place of business. However, this specific training consisted of focusing primarily on issues regarding African Americans being unfairly treated and carried a motif that Caucasian males are to blame for an inequality expressed in the vocational realm and alludes to this being the only prejudice existing in society. Not only was this a form of racism in itself, but it was also an attempt to indoctrinate citizens to line up and believe the agenda that is being presented is actually factual. In reality, there has been and continues to be inequality in the country both in and out of the workplace but there is no one race that is solely affected and so there should not be biased training that states anything other than this fact. This is but a simple example of how media manipulation and government censorship are corroding the societies of free nations. An intellectual movement known as "Critical race theory" is being taught throughout American schools and it is found at the basis of the aforementioned trainings. Scientist and people of any scholarly community, observe facts and study definitions before making reports. In keeping with this practice, I will share how one source define critical race theory:

"Critical race theory (CRT) is an intellectual movement and loosely organized framework of legal analysis based on the premise that race is not a natural, biologically grounded feature of physically distinct subgroups of human beings but a socially constructed (culturally invented) category that is used to oppress and exploit people of color. Critical race theorists hold that the United States are inherently racist insofar as they function to create and maintain social, economic, and political inequalities between whites and nonwhites, especially African Americans." (Britannica, 2021)

When considering this definition, the actions of the government, the various CRT factions, and educators in the U.S., this theory is even being abused. It is rudimentary for one to collectively stereotype an entire race of people based on the actions of some. It is equally simple-minded to demean an **entire race** of people while attempting to defend one's own race against **individuals within the group** of people one has stereotyped and mislabeled. In American schools, children are being brainwashed by some bias and diluted version of this theory. Students learn that pronouns are amorphous, and that most white people are racists, entitled, and economically favored over African Americans. I take great offense to this theory holding no racist hate and having spent eight years having to live with my grandparents because my parents could not afford a place of their own. I wore clothes that were passed down from older cousins and played with toys that were purchased at yard-sales or clearance shops. Poverty is something that effects people of all races and it is vastly untrue for these groups to be claiming that it favors specifically African Americans. This is offensive in itself also because there are wealthy people of every race. It is also extremely racist in itself for followers of this theory, education systems, and the government, to disseminate false information indicating that African Americans are the only race to experience racism or hate crimes. In America, in an attempt to create a massive diversion, mass media has constructed a mirage of manipulation that creates an image where there is only crimes and unfair treatment against African Americans, LGBTQ members, and non-male genders. Any educated person, no matter his or her race, sexual orientation, or gender, knows that this is not reality. One such theory may have held validity during the apartheid in South Africa or during the segregation in the U.S., but it is not the case today. It is unfair to the people and particularly to the children of today, for the government to be indoctrinating them with lies that will inevitably lead to a greater division between Caucasians and African Americans, homosexuals and heterosexuals, men, and women.

A sailor in the United States Navy, I was ordered to participate in and watch a DOD mandated training founded on this exact theory. The room was filled with both white people and African Americans, none of which express unfair treatment or hate towards the other. At no point in my entire career in or out of the military, did I experience a Caucasian male receiving better pay, promotion, or opportunity than an African American, homosexual, or women. In fact, when I was in high school, my football coach pulled my brother and I out of the game because he said that the African American students needed to play more than we did. A cabal of African American teammates proceeded to then mock and insult us because of our race by saying things such as,

HOW A SINGLE VIRUS BROUGHT HUMANITY TO ITS KNEES

"You'll never be as fast as *one of us* (I will not write how he referred to himself), you're just a slow and less athletic cracka' and you are right where you belong, on the bench."

Anyone who tries to tell me that racism or prejudice is a problem exclusively for African Americans, homosexuals, or women, will meet great opposition. Racism is a problem for both African Americans and Caucasians, prejudice is a problem for both homosexuals and heterosexuals and both men and women, and that is how it should be presented to the youth and to citizens. This theory of disproving the existence of *race* is not about this at all. In fact, by the nature of these trainings and indoctrinations, it is meant to cause strife, caste blame, and create negative and stereotypical beliefs about particularly white heterosexual males. If this were proper social science, it would naturally visit facts gathered from both races, all orientations, and genders. A consensus would therefore be made based on these facts, evidenced by society, that there are racist people who are Caucasian and there just as many racist people who are African American. It is a travesty to be brainwashing a nation and the world into believing anything other than this truth. Facts do not lie…people lie.

From afar, zirconium looks like diamond. Some of what you hear or see all over media may appear to be true. However, step back and assess. If it is possible to morph an image of an obese person into a supermodel figure, you would be stupid to think that there is not a myriad of other methods of disinformation and falsification that are being used by mass media. Research and investigate the information that the influencers and media you tune into share before you let your mind lazily accept it as truth. The world is overflowing with disinformation that subliminally promotes bogus or clandestine agendas. Some of these ideals may instill fear and get your heart racing but take the time to bring it into question and measure it against the known facts. If you want to purchase some expensive jewelry, you will never hand over $20,000 for an item that you have not first seen the documentation proving its validity. So why do you often spend your precious time entrusting stories that you have not been shown any evidence suggesting that they are true?

Fear is a pedestal to powerlessness. Last I checked, it was not the mass media, W.H.O., CDC, or the world governments, who gave you a call or brought you some soup when you were sick. It is the media's job is to disseminate information, and to do so with zero regard to the common people. Relax, stay healthy, and stay informed with the facts. Put your trust in the sources that have proven to be true and not in entities that have proven to be amorphous.

I am sure mostly everyone has heard of the Harvard University School of Business. There is an article written by Peter Vanderwicken called "*Why the News Is Not the Truth,*" that professionally supports the claim that media and politicians are as fallacious as the Great Oz. In this article, Vanderwicken begins,

"The U.S. press, like the U.S. government is a corrupt and troubled institution. Corrupt not so much in the sense that it accepts bribes but in a systemic sense. It fails to do what it claims to do, what it should do, and what society expects it to do."

There is universal rule throughout the world that goes something like this: *Treat others how you wish to be treated and always be true to your word.* Well, from personal experience, I completely concur with what Vanderwicken articulates in the opening of this article. Now that it has been established that the government often fails to follow this golden rule and is all too often found to be corrupt, we can delve into how this relates to the mass media. For readers around the world, I place the primary focus on the United States because of its political relevance and influence throughout the world. To convey how the governments corruption puppeteers the mass media, Vanderwicken continues,

"The news media and the government are entwined in a vicious circle of mutual manipulation, mythmaking, and self-interest. Journalists need crises to dramatize news, and government officials need to appear to be responding to crises. Too often, the crises are not really crises but joint fabrications. The two institutions have become so ensnared in a symbiotic web of lies that the news media are unable to tell the public what is true, and the government is unable to govern effectively." (From the thesis advanced by Paul H. Weaver, a former political scientist at Havard University, journalist at *Fortune Magazine*, and corporate communications executive at Ford Motor Company, in his analysis entitled *News and the Culture of Lying: How Journalism Really Works*)

Turn your eyes away from the telescopic view of your celestial horoscope for a moment and proffer your attention to a microscopic view of the media and the government actions surrounding the COVID-19 pandemic. Like the moon has an effect on the tides and so therefore controlling over 70% of the planet's surface, the political and economic environment in the United States, greatly influences most of the world. It is for this very reason, that anyone who wishes to escape manipulation and to find truth, needs to consider the following notions.

- What was the political environment in the United States like before the COVID-19 outbreak? Sure, people around the world disliked Trump and his tweets, but was there really any real unrest worthy of mass medias intervention? Not until the U.S. election grew nearer did civil unrest begin to really unfold. Take the George Floyd murder for example and the birth of the BLM movement, ANTIFA, and the mass riots and destructions that followed immediately after. George Flyod did not deserve to be murdered but he was also not a standup citizen as media blithely suggests. He was convicted of eight crimes to include aggravated robbery during a home invasion. However, he had long served his time in prison and officer Chauvin had absolutely no business murdering a free man and abusing his power as a law enforcement officer. The major issue with this situation is not even the murder itself, for justice was served and ex-officer Chauvin has been convicted of the crime. An even greater issue at hand is the media's mass production of coverage solely expressing civil unrest towards the African American community. To make matters even worse, the mass media has created civil distrust and stereotyping towards the entire law enforcement bodies nationwide. Crimes to include even murder, committed by members claiming to be a part of ANTIFA and BLM, have been ignored or simply swept under the rug instead of broadcasted in the same way the stories of officer abuse against African Americans have and continue to be. It is inarguable that the government and media are intentionally withholding crimes committed by certain groups and deliberately sharing only those committed by Caucasians (primarily associated with President Trump) or police. There is an agenda behind every news story or article and one of the reasons this has been ongoing is because the government desires for there to be a greater civil divide amidst its populations. Republicans argue that this is being done in order to secure the votes in major cities, where the population is predominately lower class and either politically liberal or democratic. Democrats simply point the finger at President Trump, his supporters, and Caucasian heterosexual males within the middle class or above. Both arguments can be viewed and both perspectives can be understood.

There are some aspects of each case that can be proven true such as the populations in major cities coincidentally being predominately African American, minorities, and Democrats, while many supporters of President Trump have proven to be extremely conservative and coincidentally Caucasian and outside the major cities. However, all of the issues surrounding these politics are meant to distract from a bigger and far more secret agenda held by our government.

While rioters are burning police vehicles and marching against the existence of police in general, the political shadows avoid the sunlight. Evidence of faulty voting machines, ballots casted by long deceased individuals and illegal immigrants, were all discovered. However, when questioned by neutral parties or by the then standing President, Donald Trump, all investigations were silenced by mass media as quickly as they had once emerged. Before President Biden or Vice President Harris had ever officially or legally taken office, mass media began blasting the world with celebratory articles of victory for African Americans, LGBTQ members, Democrats, Women, and anti-Trump supporters. One particular article read: *Congratulations to Americas first African American and first Female Vice President.* By this point in time, it was far to early for these banners for the all-holy donkey to be flown. However, by releasing this information early, media was able to stir more civil unrest and create a media blizzard so thick, all stories or actions of an investigation became invisible. America broke into chaos and Washington knew that at this point, even if an investigation had ended with President Biden and Vice President Harris being found guilty, overturning the announcements would cause further chaos throughout the country.

Coincidentally, a random riot of "Trump Supporters" stormed the capital building after a suspicious bus arrived in front of the White House. In 1814, British troops had successful invaded and destroyed the White house. Since that date centuries ago, no such invasion has ever been successful or even deemed possible. In keeping with a politically unbiased theme, I will ask this simple question: how is it possible for a group of unarmed civilians to successful invade and overtake the capital building conveniently during the most controversial election in American history, when actual militias had failed on numerous occasions since 1814? The White House is one of the most armed and protected facilities in the world. The only rational reason that civilians were able to storm the White House, was because it was all premeditated.

- On January 20th, 2021 President Joseph Biden was sworn into offer by U.S. Chief of Justice John Roberts. That same month, another reported surge of COVID-19 cases and deaths in the Continental United States hits the media front. Fauci terrifies the population and mass media shares hyperbolized accounts of massive graves in Italy and amassing death ravaging across Europe. The actual numbers that the W.H.O. and media had broadcasted to the public at this time were drastically higher than they were during the U.S. lockdowns. Meanwhile, in Europe and particularly Italy, there was never any evidence proving mass graves were being used or that death had overtaken the EU populations. In fact, by this point in time, numbers had been declining since the onset and first European lockdown. This is a very bluntly obvious example of media deception.

- Finally, members of the medical community come forth with evidence of COVID-19 number manipulation and fraudulent reporting. Instead of denying the obvious blunder or admitting its mistake, W.H.O. and the CDC used mass media to justify its miscalculations by stating that these exaggerations were estimations made in order to protect the public health. Let it be known that these miscalculations included bribing and incentivizing doctors and hospitals to exaggerate the number of cases. One way in which these entities had accomplished these manipulations was by counting almost any cause of death as being ultimately caused by COVID-19. In some cases, entire nursing homes where residents were already known to have been terminal, were including in the CDC and W.H.O. COVID-19 case and death reports. Some other causes of death that were falsely identified and reported as being COVID-19 include the following: pneumonia, heart disease, cancer, influenza, and natural death.

Although the ultimate scheme at hand is still unknown, it is definitely underway, and COVID-19 is merely a single piece of the pie. Tensions continue to rise between the United States and its enemies such as Iran and Syria. Fellow superpowers China and Russia have also expressed extreme distaste towards the U.S. and its current happenings. China has moved against Taiwan while Russia encroached on Ukraine. All of these massive foreign moves have occurred while the U.S. and its allies were busy fussing about implementing mask policies, vaccine passports, and imbuing civil unrest and inequality. Weaver of Harvard expatiates,

"The news media and the government have created a charade that serves their own interests but misleads the public. Officials oblige the media's need for drama by fabricating crises and stage-managing their responses, thereby enhancing their own prestige and power. Journalist dutifully report those fabrications. Both parties know the articles are self-aggrandizing manipulations and fail to inform the public about the more complex but boring issues of government policy and activity. What has emerged, is a culture of lying. Which is the discourse and behavior of officials seeking to enlist the powers of journalism in support of their goals, and of journalist seeking to co-opt public and private officials into their efforts to find and cover stories of crisis and emergency response."

There has been no greater evidence of this "Culture of Lying" than the situation surrounding the COVID-19 pandemic. No one knows what to believe or whom to believe and there has been a drastic decline in people's trust in government worldwide. The only viable option to learn the truth, is to continue to ask the questions, follow the facts, and think with your own head. Follow the facts like you would follow the stars! Media is, has been, and will always be, a maze of deception leading to nothing but dead-ends and fallacy.

A Sunny Day

"When you are in the eye of the storm, you are often not aware of the whiplash around you."

Hugh Bonneville, Film Actor

There was once a story of a young boy who lived in a village where verdant hills swayed with a constant wind and where wolves never ceased to challenge the farmer's flock. What was peculiar about this situation, was how the wolves managed to attack on only odd calendar days and were only ever caught in the act by the young boy. Late one evening, when the sky was a velvet swirl of blackness and stars, the young boy dutifully obeyed his father, the farmer, and ventured outside to check up on their sheep. To the boy's terror and surprise, the alpha wolf whispered over the chilly wind in a voice like that of a demon. This young boy was too young to be considered mannish but also too old to be considered boyish. It would never do him well to lie about such a serious matter or to fabricate a tale about a whispering wolf. However, when he had rushed into his father's room to alarm him, the boy was ridiculed and called a fool. The next day, the pair had discovered that two more sheep had been stolen by the wolves. When the next odd night came, the boy again dutifully followed his father's orders and ventured outside to check on the flock. This time, the alpha wolf did not only whisper, but he also cornered the young boy. Every word that was spoken by the wolf had stabbed him with fear. In exchange for his mercy, the wolf offered the boy a deal. On every even day, the boy was instructed to cry wolf to his father who would arise and rush downstairs in an attempt to slay the robber. Each time, the wolf would wait until the odd day just as he had always done, to collect his prey. After three such occasions when the boy had cried wolf, when no such wolf had been discovered, the farmer lost all trust in the young boy's word. The

HOW A SINGLE VIRUS BROUGHT HUMANITY TO ITS KNEES

farmer continued to lose more and more sheep and the boy continued to live in fear.

To those who are not familiar with this short story, the wolf was the only character to ever get what he wanted. When it comes to the COVID-19 scenario, the government, W.H.O., CDC, Bill Gates, and the various vaccine creators represent the wolves. From the beginning, they have stolen what was the people's freedom and rights. Systematically, these entities utilized mass media manipulation to instill hysteria throughout the world. Like the boy who cried wolf, these parties, continue to change information and to fabricate false promises. In Italy for example, the form that is required for a person to move from their place of residence to the grocery or to work, had been changed four times in less than two weeks. Also evidenced in Europe, the various European leaders continue to change COVID-19 measures based upon a color scale which fluctuates on statistics that have already been proven to have been manipulated. After months of undulating policy, instruction, and levels of enforcement, the people are losing patience and trust in their leadership. In the city of Naples for example, citizens rushed the streets and rioted after leader De Luca, issued a second lockdown. By this time, the truth about the mass media manipulation had been vastly known as well as opinions gathered by basic observation. When people were authorized to move freely about, they were not seeing evidence of a pandemic where millions of people were being thrown into mass graves or overcrowding hospitals. They realized who the wolves were and that they had been fed some lies and exaggeration. Fear is still a thick fog throughout the continent but there is evidence of its thinning out as people begin to fact check the information from government and media. As evidenced in the short story of the young boy and the wolf, there is only so many times one can cry wolf before all trust in one's word is lost. There is a massive rush to disseminate unapproved and unsafe vaccines, issue unnecessary lockdowns and restrictions, and hold hysteria, because the government, W.H.O., CDC, media, and other elite party players who are a part of the grand manipulation, realize that time is running out and that they have cried wolf one too many times. If you are a doubter of this philosophy of basic fact and observation, consider the following points. If what I am bringing to your attention is not true, then why the massive push and rush? You may argue it is to cease the rise in cases and deaths. However, you can clearly see that those have not teetered in months, there is still an almost one-hundred percent recovery rate, and in places where draconian law has been lifted, life could not be better. More will be elaborated on with regards to vaccines in later chapters, but keep in mind that none of the vaccines have been approved and all of them contain synthetic constituents that are proven to prevent the human body's natural immune system from either recognizing or defending against illnesses. It takes relatively two to four years for a vaccine to complete animal testing and potentially another two of voluntary human trials, before it even graduates from an *experimental phase.* Not one, but various, different vaccines have already been administered to millions worldwide. Not even two years have transpired since the first documented case of COVID-19 in December 2019. As you can see for yourself on the W.H.O. international website or via the CDC, they intentionally accelerated the process. When it comes to medicine and especially vaccines, it is a matter of law, ethics, and human rights that these practices and trials are properly and thoroughly conducted and completed before being introduced into the public. What is even more terrifying and alarming, is how these experimental and accelerated vaccines are also being mandated or incentivized in many places and by many organizations. Mandating a human being to partake in a medical experiment is against constitutional law and fractures the basis of human rights that are meant to be protected under the European Convention on Human Rights (ECHR) and by United Nations Human Rights Council. There is no misconception that the parties who are orchestrating these infractions to human rights, know that they are doing so and therefore, realize that they must administer as many doses as possible before they are halted by a realization of the truth or policed by some external force.

HOW A SINGLE VIRUS BROUGHT HUMANITY TO ITS KNEES

Why have I chosen to use *A Sunny Day*, as the title of this chapter, when there is an obvious negative connotation thus far? Answering this question is rather simple. Like a flashlight or a lantern illuminates the way to safety, the truth will do the same. Time is life's trainer and if you are among those in the populace who entrust the government, elites, W.H.O., CDC, and mass media, then time will surely have the final say. The intention is not to dissuade your beliefs or cause you to change your stance. My only objective is to share with you the truth based on what is fact. I encourage you to fact check the facts that I present to you and I encourage it so much, that I have included a proper bibliography of all the sources I have used in my research during this writing process. Let it be known that many of these sources are from the parties in question. Heed to the wise words of C.S. Lewis,

"I believe that the sun has risen not only because I see it, but because by it I see everything else."

Fact checking is no different than removing one's hands from one's own eyes and observing the sights and sounds that surround them. A fact is like the moon at night or the sun by day. Both bodies of light illuminate everything so that we can see. If you are a person who turns on the television or who scrolls through your phone aimlessly believing and entrusting the hysteria and information that you see and hear, you are a person who pretends and chooses to be blind and deaf. Fact checks the sources and information that you glean from media and government, and perhaps, you will still stand in the belief you had first developed. But at least at that point, you would have taken the necessary step of comparing these ideas and this information with the whole picture.

It is no secret, that so many people have been kept away from family members, friends, and lovers. Over the course of this pandemic, I have had to mutually end a relationship due to the impossibility for reunion. I went well over a year without being able to return to America to see my son, family, and friends. Human beings are tribal and social by nature. It is literally ingrained in our very DNA. Please take the necessary time to acknowledge the great pain you may have rightfully experienced or be experiencing still, that comes from being forced into reclusiveness and isolation. Please take a second moment to pause and to acknowledge the great anger that may arise when or if, these draconian measures turn out to have been placed in vain or by heinous hands in an attempt to further a furtive objective. Emotions are powerful potions but are more or less, clouds, holding vast power, but remaining itinerate and passing. To feel is inevitable, but to act is necessary.

After a frustrating process of having my leave or vacation, rejected six different times and for various different reasons to include whether or not I had received the vaccine, I finally set off for America for some much-needed reunion and respite from the oppressive smog of COVID-19-Europe. Arriving to the United States from Europe was a rather smooth process since I had my negative PCR test results in-hand. However, coming back to Europe from the United States was agonizingly infuriating. An appointment needs to be made in the U.S. in order to receive a PCR test for COVID-19. This is the necessary test that is required to enter most countries. Despite my having this test and the negative results, I was not permitted to board two of my flights leading to the loss of almost $2,500, an additional twelve hours at CDG in Paris, a third COVID-19 swab, and lost luggage. When questioning the European airline, I was rudely told that all passengers were now required to present a negative Antigen test 42 hours prior to their flight. Having started my journey from across the Atlantic and arriving to Paris late, there was no possibility for any of the passengers on board to accommodate to this last-minute change in policy. I am shedding light on this personal experience, which I am sure many others have experienced similar situations, in order to express the utter disarray, prejudice, corruption, and inefficacy that is surrounding the COVID-19 pandemic and the policies therein. Facts do not lie…people lie. It is a fact that both the antigen and PCR tests, have proven to produce false results and therefore cannot be one-hundred percent trusted. It is also fact that none of the experimental-vaccines are proven or even prescribed to prevent the contraction or spread of COVID-19. For an airline or government to create mandates and measures based on a test with proven unreliability and an experimental-vaccine whose manufacturers and distributors inform, has been accelerated, not yet approved, and was not created to prevent someone from contracting or spreading the COVID-19 virus but only to lessen the severity of symptoms. No matter what side you may stand, ask your intelligent mind whether this makes much sense. If the vaccine had undergone proper processes and procedures and been proven effective at preventing and protecting against the spread of the COVID-19 virus, then mandating and requiring such a vaccine would then be justified. If either the antigen or PCR tests were proven to produce reliability in its results, it would then be justifiable for an organization or company to base its policy on such a reliable confirmation. Open the blinds and let in the light! Intentionally turn your eyes to the whole picture and evaluate what truths the light from facts brings into your reality. I promise that it will prove to be a very sunny day.

Lockdown Two & Three

"The truth is I love being alive. And I love feeling free. So if I can't have those things then I feel like a caged animal and I'd rather not be in a cage. I'd rather be dead. And it's real simple. And I think it's not that uncommon."

Angelina Jolie, Actress

In shades of perfect aqua, green, and pacific blue, Poseidon's eye opened under the Tyrrhenian Sea. For the first time in over three months, I breathed in the magical sights and sounds that only the Amalfi coast can offer. To most Europeans, the end of the first lockdown came in the middle of May 2020, and it felt better than New Years. Mass media and government had spread hysteria far and wide, causing a large portion of the population to remain indoors. Under the illusion that this would be the end of lockdowns, many people spread their wings and began to travel and enjoy life again. Before the lockdown, I was traveling to a different European city every three days. To traverse the continent and inhale its cultures was the only reason why I had agreed to take a job with an organization I had lost a lot of respect for leading up to the decision. When my ability to catch flights or hit the international highways was robbed from me, I was left with only a job I dislike and an empty house. But hope is like a ship growing out of a blue horizon and I never took my eyes off of it. For several months, Europe seemed to be surfing the COVID-19 wave and gradually blossoming into the flower of tourism it had always proven to be.

From the moment my superiors began to discuss stipulations over the possibility of a second wave of COVID-19, I knew this freedom was about to be stripped away again. Politicians and government leaders were quick to accuse the summer travels of the apparent rise in cases and deaths. No one was seeing any signs of such a thing and so brushed it off or ignored such oppressive restrictions. However, to regain control, government leaders and W.H.O. representatives developed a new theory that a majority of the cases they were referring to this time, were young people who are asymptomatic. This theory was clearly a scapegoat to prevent people from questioning authority and to recreate hysteria. From the beginning of October and into the first week of November, European nations began to systematically issue lockdown orders for the second time.

Sisyphus had managed to tip the boulder up the slope and reveled in the happiness of success once he had begun to see and feel the slope becoming the top of the mountain. Alas, as the old Greek tale continues and repeats, Sisyphus quickly lost the feeling of victory as the stone magically began to roll back down to the bottom from where he first began. This story is often used to define and depict insanity. Issuing more draconian lockdowns and measures was not effective the first time around and even caused dramatic economic injury. By issuing a second round of the same measures, government leaders become real-life examples of Sisyphus's insanity in that they are doing the same things that did not work and expecting different results.

Scientist have compared the differences between lions who are bred and raised in captivity and the lions who roam wild in Africa. Based on scientific research, lions in captivity experience morphological effects that would fatally deplete the predator's ability to survive if reintroduced into the wild. By locking the beast inside a cage or fenced-in habitat, scientist proved that not only does the lion's behavior change, but its skull also literally changes shape causing it to lose some its natural functionality. Humans are social creatures just like lions. Human beings require socialization, exercise, adventure, environmental-stimulus, fresh air, and activities that keep both the body and the mind sharpened and engaged. It is against nature and is a crime against humanity to force human beings into lockdowns. Especially when medical research confirms, 99.9% of the population faces no lethal threat. Captivity can reduce the quality of life and become a detriment to wildlife so what brilliance can be found in believing that by forcing the most intelligent living organism on the planet into a lockdown, will be beneficial or even better for health?

"There's no reason we need to lock people in their home," says Devi Sridhar, chair of global public health at the University of Edinburgh.

Despite the overwhelming amount of evidence supporting the declaration that lockdowns are not an effective or healthy answer, European leaders blew the whistle, knocked the ice cream cone out of the child's hand, and forced denizens into another lockdown. This second lockdown remained in effect throughout the holidays destroying families hopes of enjoying a warm reunion. At this time, many nations around the globe had also regressed back into lockdowns. It was not until February, that European leaders began to slowly lift lockdowns again. However, this time many nations adopted a less severe draconian measure but one that still prevented citizens from traveling outside of their region of residence. To add to the drastically ineffective and joy-sapping orders, restaurants were limited to take-away only and bars could only serve through a window. Certain establishments in Italy welcomed table seating but were limited to minimal occupancy and hours. Less than a month after European leaders lifted the second lockdown, they issued a third. There is no sense in quoting statistics or numbers at this time because as you will clearly find if one doe's one's own research, they are quicksilver and have been since the very beginning. In an article posted by the *Washington Post,* Deborah Birx, of the White House coronavirus task force responded to claims that patients who died from other causes are being included in the covid death statistics,

"Those individual's will have an underlying condition, but that underlying condition did not cause their acute death when it's related to a covid infection."

HOW A SINGLE VIRUS BROUGHT HUMANITY TO ITS KNEES

Neither Fauci or Birx ever provided physical evidence to prove Fox News's Tucker Carlson and analyst Brit Hume's claims to be false. However, it was later admitted by CDC that it had in fact "estimated" its count of covid cases and deaths and that hospitals "may have" reported patients who died of other causes such as pneumonia, as having died from COVID-19. Evidence of manipulation and fraud have been exposed in both Europe and the United States and such proof is consistent with the claims expressed herein and throughout this work. Where is the truth? The problem with being bossed around by government leaders, government funded health representatives, and their organizations, is that they control the environment by controlling the media. It is very much like trying to drive a car in a torrential rainstorm with no windshield wipers on. The people deserve nothing but the truth and sadly, the people in these places have not been getting it. Another interesting statistic is shared in the same *Washington Post* article by Aaron Blake,

"But the CDC says these data are generally incomplete, even for months. A study of 2015's data showed that "mortality data is approximately 27% complete within 2 weeks, 54% complete within 4 weeks, and at least 75% complete within 8 weeks of when the death occurred."

Based on this observation shared by Blake, the CDC subliminally admitted that it has been inflating the numbers since the beginning. How can I make such a claim? You can be a firm believer in everything Fauci and the W.H.O. have put out about COVID-19, and still not be able to prove my claim wrong. Based on the CDC itself, it takes up to 8 weeks for mortality data to be only 75% complete and this is counted per death. How in less than half of this amount of time, did the world's mass media, CDC, W.H.O., and government leaders, gather enough accurate data to promote the inordinate number of COVID-19 deaths and cases that it indeed did? The obvious answer to that question is that they lied to the populace!

In several articles about the COVID-19 pandemic in Europe, W.H.O. made claims of more than 140,000 deaths across twenty-one countries after just the first week in March 2020. How is this statistically possible given that at that time, proper testing of COVID-19 was not available, nor had it even been 8 weeks since the first cry of a surge of cases broke out from media and government sources around the world? Things simply do not add up.

Most of the world can remember watching stories on the news about military vehicles being used to transport coronavirus victims to "mass graves" which were later revealed to be normal cemeteries. The date of this story was March 19, 2020 and Italian authorities broadcasted numbers nearly reaching 3,000 deaths by this point. Again, I will restate that at this time, there was not accurate testing available or a physical way to deem all of these deaths as being COVID-19 related. It is also very important to mention that of these deaths, over 85% were said to have been 75 years of age or older. Italy is also only second to Japan for being the nation with the largest percentage of elderly adults. Of these elderly adults, most were known smokers with some rather serious preexisting health issues. Italian Ministry of health states that the country has had a relatively stable death rate throughout the twenty-first century. In both 2018 and 2019, the listed death rate in Italy was 10.5 per 1,000 residents and in 2020, it was 10.658%. For mass media to have broadcasted to the world that the Italian Ministry of Health had even called in the military to assist with burials due to so many people dying, one would think the death rate would reflect something a little more drastic than merely a 0.158% increase. Thousands of people were denied the opportunity to visit loved ones who had been taken to hospitals or were being denied hospital service for real emergencies as a result of some of the draconian measures Italy and most other countries in Europe had enacted in an almost militaristic manner. Contemplating this issue alone is extremely disheartening.

In conclusion with this point, one can clearly observe that despite the pandemic, Italy has maintained the same death rate that it had since the beginning of the twenty-first century. And that can only mean one thing…the Italian government, WHO, and mass media have also been caught in a seriously morbid lie. My specific emphasis on Italy's response and media is due to the known fact that it was the country recording the highest numbers at this time. It appears that the only nations that are producing false reports are nations with close ties to the United States, which as several points from earlier chapters proved, have been lying from the beginning about COVID-19 metrics.

Florida: A Movement?

"We must have the acuity to assess whether our approach is working and know when it's time to change our approach."

Tony Robbins

All around the world, members of an unknown shadow-work, are effortfully removing, censoring, and labeling, any article or study that opposes the ideas or statistics that the government, mass media, W.H.O., and CDC, are presenting. This is a major attempt to disinform the population by working to ensure that one party maintains complete control over what information is available and what information is not. Fortunately, technology is adaptable and often provides alternative ways to share and view information that is censored or blocked. In the information technology field, we sometimes like to refer to these as *backdoors*. One such method that is commonly used to accomplish these types of operations is through the use of a personally controlled domain. Another way is through the use of applications such as *Telegram*. Of course, there exist IT professionals whose skills and know-how are far superior to my own, who could show you several other ways of accomplishing such tasks. It is to this adaptability, that I owe a great debt. Many thanks to the loyal friends, fellow truth-seekers, and fact-checkers, for sharing so many of the credible sources I am using to complete this work of truth. A normal person would naturally find a way to overcome an obstacle if they really needed to accomplish something. The COVID-19 pandemic is certainly one great obstacle that the whole world wants to overcome. Influenza is truly a terrible issue and one that proves to be year after year. Although, it takes about the same amount of lives each year consistently and it is almost exclusively, the elderly, who pass away as a result of its symptoms. When evaluating the COVID-19 situation as a whole, the real obstacles rise to the surface. It is not whether the virus is as deadly as mass media and world government proclaims, but whether these leaders have effectively and honestly responded to this public health crisis. There is a plethora of evidence validating the invalidity of media and government reports of the number of cases and mortality rates in any given location. Putting this to the side for a moment; government response to the pandemic has proven to be as exaggerated as its reports. Luckily, there are a few stubborn nations that acted directly opposite of the rest of the world from the very beginning. These nations are Sweden, Japan, South Korea, and Tajikistan. Are these nations on to something or has the decision to reject the idea of lockdowns and draconian law, cost them dearly? Learn the facts, and then you tell me.

One of the most impressive archipelagoes in the entire world, Sweden's capital city of Stockholm, is featured in a myriad of posts depicting Swedes happily sipping cafes and dining at tables together. One sign posted outside a restaurant on Drottninggatan (Queen Street), Stockholm's busiest street, reads *I ASSURE YOU WE'RE OPEN*. Children from preschool to the age of 16 were permitted to continue going to school and most businesses continued as normal but urged employees to be chary about hygiene. There were no reports of long ques of customers waiting to enter groceries or shops. The only somewhat stringent measures were placed on the elderly population because of the 2,900 deaths that were recorded by the end of May 2020, 65% were 70-75 years of age and 35% were from 80 years of age or older. It is for this statistical fact, Sweden found it unnecessary to oppress the rest of the population which experienced no deaths for that entire period. Makes a lot of sense to me. To expound even further, consider this mortality rate in comparison with a city of equal size in the United States. Over the exact same period of time, New York City recorded 18 thousand deaths with a population of 9 million whereas Sweden, recorded 2,900 deaths with a population of 10 million. Not only does Sweden have a slightly greater population than New York City, its ratio per capita is exponentially less and this is with the country having placed zero of the extreme lockdowns and measures seen in almost every other country in the world. Firstly, this proves that there is evidence that herd immunity is more effective than draconian law, including lockdowns, at preventing the spread of the COVID-19 virus. Just to name a few more examples, the state of New Jersey reported 8,549 deaths with a population of 8.8 million people while the state of New York reported 25 thousand deaths with a population of 19 million people. Even when these ratios are expressed on a larger scale, they are still showing results that are significantly worse. Again, further proving that the general response taken by most of the world, was not the correct one.

According to WebMD, Herd Immunity, "is when a large part of the population of an area is immune to a specific disease. If enough people are resistant to the cause of a disease, such as a virus or bacteria, it has nowhere to go. Herd immunity protects at-risk populations. These include babies and those whose immune systems are weak and can't get resistance on their own."

Based on the reports of death rates and the ages of those patients worldwide, there is unanimous evidence showing that the covid-19 virus, like influenza, is primarily lethal to elderly and those with underlying health conditions or malfunctioning immune systems. Taking a second glance at the definition of herd immunity, one can clearly observe that the situation surrounding the covid-19 pandemic, would call for such a response. The primary mission of this work is to provide you with the abundance of facts that can be used as water to put out those flames of fear and hysteria brought on by mass media and government. Take a breath, smile, cling to hope, and embrace life my fellow truth-seeker and fellow human.

Turning the discussion over to Japan; let it be known that the country's total population is currently 127 million people. For being a relatively small country in size, that is a rather dense populace. While Swedes were enjoying the typical Nordic chill without ever paying homage to Draco the horrible and his hackneyed draconian ways, Japanese officials and epidemiologists were responding with even less severity. As the world was approaching the summer of 2020 with caution and utter exhaustion, Japanese citizens were dancing and

HOW A SINGLE VIRUS BROUGHT HUMANITY TO ITS KNEES

having a great time in the various nightclubs throughout the country's most vibrant cities. Officials only decided to close these establishments because of the world's negative response to their far more leisureful measures against the COVID-19 virus. However, the world had no justification in bad-mouthing or judging Japan's response and methods because since the initial surge of the pandemic, the country had reported only 558 deaths in total by Summer 2020 and have maintained the slowest progression in the world to-date. Mass media and its twisted jargon, attempted to demean the success of Japanese people and leaders by trying to claim this accomplishment was only possible because of the nation's small size. In response to this gobbledygook, both officials and experts pointed out that Tokyo alone, is just as crowded, if not more crowded, than New York City. For anyone who has ever traveled to the technologically advanced and bustling city of Tokyo, entrusting such a fact should be axiomatic. Thus, Japan is just another example of the effectiveness of herd immunity against the COVID-19 pandemic. Japan also happens to be the country with the world's largest population of elderly. Fear is fire and however it is used, solely depends on the person yielding it. Facts do not lie…people lie.

By now, you should have read enough and done enough research of your own, to realize that mass media, W.H.O., CDC, and the government, do not wish to cool the flames of fear within you…they willingly wish to bellow the existing fires. For to man and woman, what greater fear is there, than the fear of the great unknown.

Close your eyes and imagine that you are waking up to a summer rainstorm. Now, try to feel the emotions that would come after experiencing only rainy and gray days over the entire summer season. Pause and begin to picture that first day when the sun makes an appearance, and the rain begins to abate. Senator Scott Jensen, M.D., Family Physician, Senator (R-Minnesota) offers factual information that can be received like sunshine after months of rain. After months of incessant monotony produced by the mass media and government leaders regarding the COVID-19 fear-factory, Senator Jensen talks to Tony Robbins about how he and the physicians across America, were incentivized by Medicare and the US government, to list any and every death, no matter what the actual cause, as ultimately being caused by COVID-19. During an interview from *The Tony Robbins Podcast*, Senator Jensen exposits,

"I think it was April 3rd, I received a communication from the state department of health and in that we were basically being advised as physicians as to how to correctly complete a death certificate if covid-19 was involved directly or perhaps, even presumptively, probably, or peripherally involved and when I read the document, I had read that there was a link for further information through the CDC. So, I went there, and I just shook my head and said, 'no, this is wrong." I just raised up the flagpole if you will, and I reached out to fifty to seventy-five physicians that I am in fairly close contact with and I am no spring chicken. I have done death certificates for some time and I have never been coached or massaged in this way. I was coached and massage to utilize covid-19 as a factor in the causation of death even if I had not checked a covid-19 test; even if I hadn't had an interest in one, and right around that time, Dr. Burkes from Washington D.C. said, 'Nobody's going to die with covid-19…if they have it, they're dying of it,' and that was about the silliest thing I have ever heard."

As evidenced in this interview, there are in fact, economic incentives presented to physicians and hospitals for manipulating death certificates to reflect a higher number of covid-19 deaths. Senator Jensen had even begun to share his findings of the corruptions being committed by U.S. government, W.H.O., CDC, and most world leaders, but was quickly met with backlash from even American people who he said, "seemed not to be interested in facts." USA Today conducted a fact check on Senator Jensen's findings and had even concluded that his numbers were in fact, true at proving the manipulations were being made. It goes without saying, the nurses, physicians, scientist, and everyone, who have honestly been working around

HOW A SINGLE VIRUS BROUGHT HUMANITY TO ITS KNEES

the clock to fight this pandemic and help people, deserve nothing but respect and gratitude. None of these professionals have done anything but sacrifice their own time and health to serve the people. You are all truly amazing and I thank you from the bottom of my heart no matter where in the world you may be serving. As for the government leaders and organizations who have proven to be less than honest, to you, I earnestly expose your shameful actions and pray that the truth finds its way in front of billions of eyes.

Within the United States, there have been two states that have stepped out and opposed the governments and worlds draconian responses. Florida is home to some of the most beautiful beaches in the world which is one reason why I was not at all surprised when I saw a news story showing crowds of smiling faces enjoying the sunshine and fraternization. It was disheartening to see headlines from media around the world, ridiculing these people for being people. Florida was one of the first states to turn away from the lockdowns and closures being prescribed to people throughout the world. There are too many physicians, pathologist, immunologist, virologist, epidemiologist, scientist, infectious disease experts, around the world, to name, who have proudly and bravely come forward to oppose the lies being broadcasted by mass media about covid-19 by sharing professional facts. In light of facts uncovered by credible sources from the front lines, Florida Governor Ron DeSantis told the world that he did not want to,

"hurt families who can't afford to shelter in place for six weeks, especially not for a virus that has a 99.8 percent survival rate." (WPEC)

Florida residents are not required to wear facial masks of any kind and there are currently no restrictions limiting basic operation. For the United States, it seems like Gov. DeSantis started a small movement that attracted the attention of some other state officials and people throughout the nation.

According to the *Texas Tribune*, Texas Governor Greg Abbott told reporters,

"There won't be any more lockdowns in the state. I want to focus on working to heal those who have covid-19 so they can leave the hospitals and get back to their normal routines."

In an Executive Order by the state of Texas, Gov. Abbott ordered an official reopening of businesses with no covid-19 related operating restrictions, lifted mask requirements, and strongly encouraged state residents to practice good-faith efforts to keep case numbers low. This Executive Order was established on March 02, 2021.

Arguably the most substantial case against the government, W.H.O., and CDC recommendations for COVID-19 response, came from South Dakota Governor, Kristi Noem. On Twitter, she wrote,

"We already know that lockdowns DON'T stop the spread of the virus. However, they destroy small businesses and jobs, and they make it difficult for families to put food on the table."

Also, when questioned by the nation's medical representatives about the rise of cases in her state being caused by her refusal to put in place mask mandates, she responded,

"That is not true. There are 41 states that have some kind of a mask mandate. Cases are on the rise in 39 of those 41 states. Now some in media are saying that South Dakota is the worst in the world right now and that is absolutely false."

I am in full support of Gov. Noem's declarations and her refusal to put the people of her state at an economical loss when statistical evidence shows her actions have made little to no difference to the numbers or to the overall wellbeing of her residents. Likewise, Florida and Texas have bravely stepped forward towards the truth and towards normalcy. As the month of April 2021 ended, Tennessee became the next state to officially order a lift on all COVID-19 related bans and restrictions. It is only by prayer and hope, that the other 46 states quickly follow suit.

HOW A SINGLE VIRUS BROUGHT HUMANITY TO ITS KNEES

There is a lot of power in being able to walk in the opposite direction of friends and comfort when you realize there is something amiss. Admittedly, I approached my education with OCD-like attention and settled for nothing less than an A. This success in the classroom had at first, cost me some popularity outside of it. Alas, after receiving a written invitation to attend Dartmouth University under the funds of a scholarship, I knew I had done right to avoid the excessive frivolity that was so commonly expressed among my peers. I guess you could argue that going against the grain became sort of habit of mine. At the rise of COVID-19, I refused to swallow the cool-aid full of fear juice. Once mask mandates were set into place, I was always sliding mine off of my face to ensure that I kept my cortisol levels low and my intake of fresh air, high. In the world of fitness, high cortisol levels weaken the immune system, induce stress, alter mood, inhibit muscle growth, and can ultimately lead to more serious health issues such as Cushing syndrome. Rapid or interfered breathing, such as the kind experienced while wearing a face mask, can cause an increase of stress levels in the body which trigger atypical synthesis from a combination of glands referred to as the HPA axis. An elite trainer and fitness nutrition specialist who has years of education and practice, I can confidently share that it is often common for fitness members wishing to either burn fat or build lean muscle mass, to supplement cortisol blockers into their diet. During an extremely stressful time in my life, I had experienced some of the negative effects of high cortisol levels to include weakened muscles and depression. To combat this issue, I consumed a cortisol blocker called *AfterGlow*, which was a product that used to be sold by BioRhythm. Having done my research prior and after confirming my findings with my physician, I was not surprised once the decreased cortisol levels alleviated my symptoms. Breathing irregularities such as tachypnea or rapid breathing, are very common side effects that people are struggling with around the world from wearing face masks for extended periods of time. It should be known that this is but one of many negative aspects to prolonged mask wearing.

PUBLIC ENEMY #1: COVID-19

As a teenager, I would sometimes accompany my stepdad during one of his construction jobs where he would often provide me with my own face mask to wear while we were working with certain materials such as paint or fiberglass. I remember reading a small note on the exterior of the mask stating that it was not meant for prolonged use. I also remember my stepfather reminding me to take periodic breaks to exit the space and breathe some fresh air. Facemasks are commonly used by individuals in various different industries including medicine. Contrary to what many of us are told, even surgeons admit to needing to step aside and catch a few breaths of fresh air during unusually long surgeries. Former member of the Cardiovascular Division and Veterans Affairs Palo Alto Healthcare System at Stanford University, Baruch Vainshelboim, constructed a hypothesis arguing against the effectiveness of wearing a facemask to prevent the transmission of the COVID-19 virus. In his research, he provides the following findings:

"The physical properties of medical and non-medical facemasks suggest that facemasks are ineffective to block viral particles due to these differences in scales. According to the current knowledge, the virus SARS-CoV-2 has a diameter of [60nm to 140 nm (nanometers billionth of a meter)], while medical and non-medical facemasks' thread diameter ranges from [55 to 440 (micrometers one millionth of a meter)], which is more than 1000 times larger. Due to the difference in sizes between SARS-CoV-2 diameter and facemasks thread diameter (the virus is 1000 times smaller), SARS-CoV-2 can easily pass through any facemask. The efficiency filtration rate falls to 15% and 58% while using surgical and N95 medical facemasks, respectively when even a small gap between the mask and the face exists."

Based on these scientific metrics, the government, CDC, and W.H.O., have also exaggerated the effectiveness of wearing a facemask. At the beginning of the pandemic, the WHO stated, "facemasks are not required, as no evidence is available on its usefulness to protect non-sick persons and cloth or gauze mask are not recommended under any circumstance."

To offer the public more confusion, the WHO made later statements promoting the effectiveness of both cloth and gauze masks and even encouraged both members who expressed symptoms and those who were healthy, to don them in order to prevent the spread of the virus. The WHO contradicts itself again by making a third statement which contradicts the second by stating that only those who are infected or who are expressing symptoms should wear cloth or gauze masks while individuals who are asymptomatic, should refrain from wearing these masks. I was definitely alive and well for the entire duration of the COVID-19 pandemic and I clearly remember the worldwide confusion about mask mandates and effectiveness. Military members were ordered to cut up segments of their uniforms and instructed on how to then create a mask out of the material. The U.S. government failed to provide its service members with masks until long after the first lockdown had ended. It was not until the timeframe during the issuance of the second lockdown in Europe, that U.S. servicemembers received the order to wear only N95 masks and informed that cloth masks were no longer authorized or effective. The WHO's stance and lack of evidence revolving around the effectiveness of wearing a facemask to prevent the spread of COVID-19, is extremely contradicting and inconsistent.

Whether you are among the fortunate few who live in either Florida, Texas, South Dakota, Tennessee, Japan, or Sweden, or you are among the majority of the world, where you have been stuck in a place with little to no relief from extreme restrictions, you need to be exposed to the truth. We are all in this together no matter what the final outcome may bring. At the end of the day, it is all about the individual being properly informed so that the individual has the opportunity to make sound decisions about their own health, politics, and public safety.

HOW A SINGLE VIRUS BROUGHT HUMANITY TO ITS KNEES

Vaccine Banter & Release

"If everything's the same, then there aren't any choices! I want to wake up in the morning and decide things!"

Lois Lowry, *The Giver*

During an interview with a panel of 7 highly qualified researchers, an experienced epidemiologist, a Nobel Laureate, and M.D.'s testing and treating patients on the frontlines, Tony Robbins, compares the way mass media and government is trying to shut down all risk, to a person deciding to drive a car every day. He goes on to explain,

"1.25 billion people die every year in car accidents. That is 3,200 people a day, every single day, around the world. If all day long, you watched the news and they showed every car accident, every person dying, you would be completely overwhelmed, you would not get into your car. And yet today, most of us drive down the street and how do we do it knowing there is nothing but a yellow line dividing us; all these crazies; some are gonna go to sleep, some who are texting, are gonna kill someone, some who are drunk are gonna kill someone, 3,200 times a day all over the earth and yet people still get into their cars and drive. It is because no one is telling you all day long what your risk is. And because you use the *F-word*, faith, to say, 'I have certainty within me that if I stay home, I have no life. So, of course I am going to drive down the street even though I could die, and I know people do die and the ratios are even smaller with COVID-19."

Tony makes an excellent point here to emphasize that there is no possibility for a life without risk. The world governments and media are instilling an unhealthy hysteria that inarguably goes against natural life. As Tony stated, people make the decision to take a calculated risk even when they get inside their car and drive to work every day. Possessing the freedom and ability to make your own decisions about how you spend your day or whether you want to take a certain risk or not, is one of the most powerful aspects of humanity. In recent world politics, the issue of abortion is being widely contested. On one side of the argument, women are demanding the freedom to choose whether to have an abortion or not and deem the governments intervention on this issue, an abuse to their individual freedom of choice over their own body. This leads to a discussion about human rights and a person's freedom of health.

Consuming too much alcohol can lead to fatal diseases like cirrhosis of the liver. Despite the proven risks to one's health, alcohol can freely be purchased and consumed in quantities and in frequencies, of an individual's choosing. A doctor may inform a person of their condition but that doctor and that person's government, has no legal right to stop that person from consuming anymore alcohol. It may be in the WHO's heart to really help society to overcome the COVID-19 pandemic. However, it is not within its rights, to intervene on a person's decision whether to take an experimental vaccine. By law, the government has the authority to issue draconian-style measures on its people, if and when it is executed in the name of public health or safety. In the chapters leading up to this one, several cases of evidence are provided that would prove that the COVID-19 pandemic was never an emergency or lethal enough threat, for governments to justify its execution of such draconian methods. This chapter is solely bent on focusing on an even greater crime against humanity and abuse of individual freedom of health.

In the beginning of December this past year, two variations of an experimental vaccine for COVID-19 were administered to the public for the first time. The release of these initial versions of the vaccine gradually became available in countries around the world. In March of 2020, Dr. Fauci told the American people and the entire listening world, that there was no such thing as a deployable vaccine in less than twelve to eighteen months. This was but one of the many ploys of fear mongering used by media, Dr. Fauci, the WHO,

CDC, and a majority of the world's government officials. It is important that the world is reminded of this statement in particular and of these facts. In less than nine months from the onset of COVID-19, these drug companies are injecting the world populace with an unapproved and improperly tested vaccine. An accelerated release, justified by a political banner claiming that it is a necessary form of emergency response. According to the CDC's own vaccine testing and approval process, there are several stages of the development cycle of a vaccine that clearly state the necessity of completion in full before public dissemination. On the CDC's official website, the stages are clearly listed to include both the duration periods of each stage and the processes within each. These general stages are used as guidelines and law for the WHO and medical science worldwide. The stages of development of new vaccines are as follows (CDC.gov, 2021):

1. Exploratory stage
2. Pre-Clinical Stage
3. Clinical Stage
4. Regulatory Review and Approval
5. Manufacturing
6. Quality Control

As stated by the WHO and CDC, the clinical development alone, consists of a three-phase process and is described by CDC verbatim:

"During Phase 1 (Of clinical Stage/Phase 3 of whole process), small groups of people receive the trial vaccine. In Phase 2, the clinical study is expanded, and vaccine is given to people who have characteristics (such as age and physical health) similar to those for whom the new vaccine is intended. In Phase 3, the vaccine is given to thousands of people and tested for efficacy and safety. Many vaccines undergo Phase 4 formal, ongoing studies after the vaccine is approved and licensed. For more information and to find out about new vaccines on the horizon, see the World Health Organization's (WHO's) Development of New Vaccines web page."

It is a proven fact, that the release of the various trial vaccines for the COVID-19 virus in response to the world pandemic goes against this very doctrine and law. Such an action against the safety of public health, was only permitted by the authority and decision of government and world leaders such as Dr. Fauci with WHO. Based on WHO and CDC guidelines, this meticulous and intentionally lengthy process and procedure is meant to ensure public safety remains the top priority. Under no conditions, is a worldwide and accelerated release of trial vaccines to the general public, safe or aligned with protecting basic human rights. The College of Physicians of Philadelphia state,

"Vaccine development is a **long**, **complex** process, often lasting **10-15 years** and involving a combination of public and private involvement," and elaborate on each phase of development in detail based on credible medical and scientific sources, with a collective and unanimous understanding. At the first set stage or phase of the vaccine development process,

"federally funded academic and governmental scientists identify natural or synthetic antigens that might help prevent or treat a disease. These antigens could include virus-like particles, weakened viruses, or bacteria, weakened bacterial toxins, or other substances derived from pathogens."

The duration of this first phase is between 2-4 years and consists of laboratory research and animal studies. Phase 2 or the second stage of the vaccine development process is known as the "Pre-Clinical Stage," and according to scientific and medical experts,

"Pre-clinical studies use tissue-culture or cell-culture systems and animal testing to assess the safety of the candidate vaccine and its immunogenicity, or ability to provoke an immune response. Animal subjects may include mice and monkeys. These studies give researchers an idea of the cellular responses they might expect in humans. They may also suggest a safe starting dose for the next phase of research as well as a safe method of administering the vaccine.

Researchers may adapt the candidate vaccine during the pre-clinical state to try to make it more effective. They may also do challenge studies with the animals, meaning that they vaccinate the animals and then try to infect them with the target pathogen.

Many candidate vaccines **never progress beyond this stage because they fail to produce the desired immune response…and usually involves private industry."**

The duration of this second stage, is an additional 1-2 years from the time of completion of phase 1. After learning about only two of this sometimes, 4-stage process, we have gleaned from credible sources such as the CDC, WHO, medical epidemiologists and experts in infectious disease, that these two phases alone, would take a minimal of 3 years to complete and verify before being passed to phase 3.

When pharmaceutical research and development companies such as Pfizer and Moderna handed out their unapproved but emergency-permitted trial vaccines as if they were candy bars on Halloween, they had skipped years of trials and procedures and the verifying results therein, that are unquestionably vital for ensuring the safety of the world's populace and proving the long- or short-term efficacy and safety of the vaccine. Therefore, it is both a medical and scientific fact that none of the vaccines that are being administered to the world's population, can offer the veracious assurances involving any of the following: safety of the vaccine, drug interactions, effectiveness of vaccine at dampening symptoms, success of vaccine at preventing transmission and therefore, lowering the number of cases and infection-rates, known long term side-effects such as infertility (none proven because proper testing was bypassed), side-effects in cases involving age or preexisting health conditions, effects on women who are pregnant, or any other vaccine-to-human effectuality that would have otherwise, been either validated and discovered or unvalidated, during the normal periods and durations of vaccine development and trialing; processes strictly and wholly meant to ensure a vaccine product is safe for public use and that anyone partaking in its use, is confidently and factually made aware of the integrity, interactions, side-effects, and trial results of said vaccine product. Adherence to these vaccine development and vaccine assurance processes is legally required by WHO/CDC, U.S. and EU Government, and the European Medicines Agency (EMA). Only because these agencies either altered or added exceptions in the last six months, are these agencies not being suspected or charged for breaking laws of public safety.

Maybe you are reading this after having already received one of the trial vaccines. Perhaps, you are like the greater percentage of the world population, and you had been misinformed and did not know that this injustice and crime against humanity had occurred. Maybe, you did not even know that these vaccines were not approved or if such a process even existed. Every day, I am dumbfounded by the great number of misinformed or uninformed minds. Countries like Italy, where the largest percentage of the population is elderly and not technologically equipped or inclined, mass manipulation and compliance are easy things for governments to achieve. Fear in the people proffers power to the government whereas, hope in the people hones honesty in the government. However, learning of the vast amount of misinformed or uniformed people in places with predominately younger and more technologically adroit populations such as the United States and the United Kingdom, is more astounding and gravely disappointing. Deciding whether to take a trial vaccine for a virus that is drastically proven to be non-lethal to an overwhelming percentage of the world's population, is almost nonsensical under any circumstance. You are making a decision about your health and your body, which makes it a decision that is among the most important in your life. It takes but only a moment of research to learn about any of the information I have provided especially regarding these trial vaccines. If you are a parent, would you feed your son or daughter pills provided from a stranger wearing a hood? This person could be an angelic being eager to make your child's life better. This person could also be the WHO or government, mass media or Big Pharma, who are offering a pill that may ruin your chances of ever becoming a grandparent or even rob you of your child altogether. Any and every good parent who loves their children would never take pills from a stranger regardless. A first and obvious step for you to take is to lift up the hood. In other words, **fact check**. Stop and be diligent about researching who is offering you a vaccine and what is being stated about this vaccine. The minute it takes to ask yourself these questions, to look away or turn off the mass media or government faces, and conduct simple research, is worth it if your child's life is in risk. If you are not a parent, if your own life were at risk, would you not agree that it is worth it to at least gather a better understanding from credible resources, before injecting yourself with a trial vaccine mass media and the government is **rushing** to get out? There is an old adage from the days of Ellis Island, when immigrants from Europe rushed after the *American Dream and Pursuit of Happiness*, that goes like this:

Too good is no good. Nothing that is done in haste is not a waste.

Protect your health because it is a glass ball in the hands of life while the government, work, and whatever else may be motivating you to blindly follow, is but only a ball made of rubber. If you drop the glass ball, your life is shattered into pieces and will never look the same, if you are even able to attach some of those broken pieces back together. Drop the rubber ball, and it will bounce back into your hands as quickly as you dropped it. **Facts do not lie…people lie.**

If the trial vaccines had underwent the proper processes and achieved positive results in effectivity and safety within the laboratory and with animals, they would have then had to proceed with a series of clinical trials to involve testing on humans but only to those who offer their voluntarily consent. This part of the process is knowns as phase 3 or stage 3, which is broken down into three to four subphases. Experts proffer a clear and precise outline of this process:

"The first attempt to assess the candidate vaccine in humans involves a small group of adults, usually between 20-80 subjects. If the vaccine is intended for children, researchers will first test adults, and then gradually step down to the age of the test subjects until they reach their target. Phase 1 trials may be non-blinded (also known as open label in that the researchers and perhaps subjects know whether a vaccine or perhaps placebo is used).

The goals of Phase 1 testing are **to assess the safety of the candidate vaccine and to determine the type and extent of immune response that the vaccine provokes.** A promising Phase 1 trial will progress to the next stage."

Phase 2 of the clinical vaccine trials will be conducted with a larger group of subjects. It is for this very reason, that evidence is produced proving that the trials that had been conducted during the first phase had proven to be successful with a smaller group of subjects well before graduating to phase 2, where a larger group of subjects will be tested. Vaccine and disease experts continue,

"A larger group of several hundred individuals participate in Phase 2 testing. Some of the individuals may belong to groups at risk of acquiring the disease. These trials are randomized and well controlled and include a placebo group. The goals of Phase 2 testing are to study the candidate vaccine's safety, immunogenicity, **proposed dosses, schedule of immunizations, and method of delivery.**"

The sentence that has been bolded, emphasizes on the fact that this phase 2 of the phase 3 clinical vaccine trials, is the step where scientist and experts determine the dosage, schedule, and method of delivery for the vaccine. Considering that all of the trial vaccines that have been mass produced and distributed, have bypassed this entire phase as well as some of the phases before it, and while it is clearly stated that the fulfillment of each phase is to be chronologically and sequentially essential before deeming a vaccine product to be safe for mass production and public dispensing, it is impossible for us common people to know whether in fact it is either beneficial or dangerous to receive two dosages of the trial vaccine or whether there is validity in the periods of time between each dosage that WHO and CDC have prescribed. For governments around the world to be fully aware of the great risks involved due to the bypassed processes necessary to prove the safety of these vaccine products to the public health, and to still continue to administer or sometimes to even mandate, citizens to receive these trial vaccines, is one of the largest cases of crimes against humanity to ever have occurred without alarming the world into war.

A simple question that I myself and everyone in the world, have the right to know, is why rush a process that has proven to not only be a medically and scientifically sound process but also one, that has still led to numerous occasions of recall and morbidity? Does that not confirm that the acceleration of these processes poses a greater risk to the world population than the virus itself? Why are you not following your own process to ensure safety to public health (WHO, CDC, EMA)? In a situation as serious as the one you perpetuate via every lane of mass media; it seems like it would be even more important for these processes to be carried out completely? Why rush a trial vaccine that has no evidence it works, when you can continue to test and develop a vaccine that clinically proves to be safe and effective? This whole conundrum with the release of these trial vaccines being accelerated, seems counter-productive and blatantly dangerous. It is because none of these questions are ever answered, that I believe COVID-19 to be less a biological threat, and more a political manipulation and plot against humanity and society as we know it. Only a fool attempts to cross a bridge without carefully testing each and every step.

Finally, vaccines that successfully graduate from the preliminary stages will move into the third and final stage of the clinical vaccine trials known as Phase 3 of phase 3. Physicians go on to say,

"Successful Phase 3 candidate vaccines move on to larger trials, involving thousands to tens of thousands of people. These Phase 3 tests are randomized and double blind and involve the experimental vaccine being tested against a placebo (the placebo may be a saline solution, a vaccine for another disease, or some other substance).

One Phase 3 goal is to assess vaccine safety in a large group of people. Certain rare side effects might not surface in the smaller groups of subjects tested in earlier phases. For example, suppose that an adverse event related to a candidate vaccine might occur in 1 of every 10,000 people. To detect a significant difference for a low-frequency event, the trial would have to include 60,000 subjects, half of them in the control, or no vaccine, group (Plotkin SA et al. *Vaccines,* 5th ed. Philadelphia: Saunders, 2008).

Vaccine efficacy is tested as well. These factors might include: 1) Does the candidate vaccine prevent disease? 2) Does it prevent infection? 3) Does it lead to production of antibodies or other types of immune responses related to the pathogen?"

As found on the CDC, WHO, and EMA webpages, after years of onerous trialing, testing, and reporting, a vaccine product that has proven successful through this final phase, must then undergo a process of product approval before it is made available to the public. In the case of the trial vaccines for the COVID-19, legal and fundamental steps of the development process were bypassed, and all of the normal process of product approval ignored and bypassed in its entirety. As stated by the CDC, the vaccine product approval process is referenced verbatim and a process of a similar nature, can be referenced on the EMA webpage:

"The U.S. Food and Drug Administration's (FDA's) Center for Biologics Evaluation and Research (CBER) is responsible for regulating vaccines in the United States. The sponsor of a new vaccine product follows a multi-step approval process, which typically includes:

- An Investigational New Drug application
- Pre-licensure vaccine clinical trials

- A Biologics License Application (BLA)
- Inspection of the manufacturing facility
- Presentation of findings to FDA's Vaccines and Related Biological Products Advisory Committee (VRBPAC)
- Usability testing of product labeling

After approving a vaccine, FDA continues to oversee its production to ensure continuing safety. Monitoring of the vaccine and production activities, including periodic facility inspections, must continue as long as the manufacturer holds a license for the vaccine product. FDA can require a manufacturer to submit the results of their own tests for potency, safety, and purity for each vaccine lot. FDA can require each manufacturer submit samples of each vaccine lot for testing."

By this point in your reading, I hope that you have become aware of the extensivity of the vaccine development and have a clear understanding on how important it is for a pharmaceutical company that is manufacturing a vaccine product, to follow each phase accordingly until the final phase. Evidence proving the need for proper approval and licensing of vaccine products have also been provided to you. In light of these potentially new understandings, do you agree with the government's decision to contradict these proven processes and to allow private pharma companies to begin disseminating experimental vaccines that have never undergone such tests, time, and validation? Mass media and WHO around the world are sharing reports of how successful these trial vaccines are already proving to be. I am certainly not the first soul nor the most qualified, to blow the whistle on anyone or any story making such fallacious and impossibly untrue claims. Anyone who is reading the scientific facts from experts in various qualifying fields of study and vocation that I am sharing, cannot believe these false claims either. Media and government have proven by their countless inflations of morbidity rates and death tolls, that they have interests that do not include the safety or betterment of the world populace. If they truly cared, do you not think they would have already been sharing the information and information similar in nature that I have with you, with the rest of the world? Instead, physicians, scientists, people on the front lines, fact-checkers, and truth-seekers, proved that WHO, CDC, government officials, and mass media, have been lying and continue to lie.

Dr. Fauci of WHO, has been called out for sharing false reports about COVID-19 deaths, total cases, mandates, vaccines, death rates, and has lied to the people on nearly twenty separate occasions. Dr. Fauci is an accomplished physician and acclaimed expert in epidemiology which makes his word hard to refute. It is like he merely wanted to defend his pride and position when his mistakes and lies were exposed and presented. Take for example, how during an interview in January of 2020, he urged the American people to relax and continued to downplay the severity of the then predominately foreign COVID-19 outbreak. The following month, he is on media telling people it is fine if they want to go on a cruise or on vacation. Then, in an interview to the public and via mass media, he said, "There is no such thing as a deployable vaccine in less than 12 to 18 months," which smartly aligns with the information provided by WHO about how the process for the development and approval of a vaccine alone, could take up to a decade or longer. But taking the spotlight off of a known professional physician and expert and placing it onto the mass media or pharmaceutical giants who have countlessly proven to provide incorrect information, and whom have fortunes to gain by playing to the tune of manipulation. Of course, Pfizer, AstraZeneca, Moderna, Johnson & Johnson, and various others, want governments to purchase and fund their vaccines and research. Of course, these companies do not care that they were approved to bypass years of necessary trials and testing. Media stations and journalist are in heaven. They have only to gain from the hysteria. What better way to up the ratings and increase viewers, than to bellow flames of fear and inflated stats? Every eye and ear have been turned their way. Money and power are manmade and very unreal things. They are both however, historical ingredients for genocide, disaster, and mass corruption.

HOW A SINGLE VIRUS BROUGHT HUMANITY TO ITS KNEES

Like in the United States, the European Medicines Agency, has allowed for a massive flex to occur in its normal vaccine development and approving processes. Whenever contested, the EMA along with the ETF, or COVID-19 Task Force, quickly justifies this decision to break and change policy. On the webpage, one can view a standard process for the approval of vaccines that mirrors that of the U.S. Also on this page, there are contradicting justifications throughout such as, an acceleration to the virus has not tampered the integrity of the processes effectiveness nor has it skewed the results. Claiming that because COVID-19 is a novel virus, it called for scientist and developers to develop an entirely new process for the development and approval of vaccines, COVID-19 vaccines to be specific, that fast-tracks through all phases. In confluence with the European Commission, the EMA and ETF report the following on the EMA webpage,

"According to the EU pharmaceutical legislation, the standard timeline for the evaluation of a medicine is a maximum of 210 active days. However, EMA treats marketing authorization applications for COVID-19 products in an expedited manner. This allows the timeline for evaluation to be reduced to less than 150 working days."

Before I begin to expound and elaborate on all the adverse effects that so many people worldwide have been suffering from, let me emphasize the *rush* and *flex* being allowed by the EMA just as is being seen within the CDC. When we are hurrying off to work after pressing the snooze button, we leave the house with messy hair, untidy shirt, coffee stains, and an ID left behind at home. This is a common occurrence and an understandable one. But why do we forget to accomplish these little daily tasks when we are frenetically trying to get out the door so to avoid being late for work? The answer to that question is because we find ourselves to be in a rush and when we are in a rush, we tend to forget little steps that we would have otherwise, easily accomplished! This is what is happening as a result of hysteria causing a massive rush to get a trial vaccine out and into the public. The EMA and CDC are accepting the messy hair and forgotten ID of these various vaccine producing companies and therefore, placing the entire European population at a greater risk than they would have otherwise been in, by simply facing the virus naturally. Proof of such a theory can be seen in countries like Sweden or Japan or in states like Texas, Florida, and South Dakota. What does messy hair and a forgotten ID look like when it comes to these big pharma companies? By allowing itself to rush its own processes and procedures out of pointless and unfounded fear, the EMA and CDC have experienced recalls of trial vaccines from several of these big pharma companies to include AstraZeneca, Moderna, Pfizer, and Johnson & Johnson.

Maybe you have returned to the store and learned that one of your favorite supplements had been recalled; so, what! In a simple scenario like this, it is not such a big deal to have an item be recalled. However, in the predicament involving the trial vaccines from these various pharma companies, the EMA, and CDC, these vaccines are being recalled due to large numbers of people who are either experiencing side effects, interactions, or death as a result of receiving said vaccine. If the EMA and CDC and the comparable government medical agencies around the world had not rushed the vaccine-train along the tracks, they would have discovered these reactions or the potentiality of them occurring, during the preliminary phases and over the prescribed window of time that it takes to properly observe subjects and results.

A litany of countries around the world from Australia to the United Kingdom, have reported cases of blood clots and deaths caused by thrombotic anomalies in patients who had received the AstraZeneca trial vaccine. Between 6 to 13 days after receiving the Johnson & Johnson vaccine, The Vaccine Adverse Event Reporting System (VAERS) had reported deaths caused from thrombotic anomalies. In these patients, of which a majority were women ranging in age from 18 and 48, the victims were otherwise clinically healthy. The Advisory Committee on Immunization Practices (ACIP) has tirelessly been evaluating this situation along with the CDC. Countless numbers of people who have received the J&J variation of the experimental vaccine, have also reported having experienced shortness of breath, horrible headaches, abdominal pain, leg pain, and several other mild to severe reactions. When questioned about these reports and reminded that the trial vaccine proved to be only 85% effective against preventing infectious disease during accelerated testing, Dr. Papa on Johnson & Johnson responded by saying,

"Those aren't the numbers that matter. What matters is how well the vaccines protect against serious disease. You still have to wear a mask and stay socially distant to protect other people-but you're free."

According to the CDC and WHO, the effectiveness of the COVID-19 vaccines is being measured by how well the vaccine proves to prevent **any infectious disease** not just COVID-19. So based upon this statement, are they telling people that these shots are no different than an influenza shot most had already received and whether one is vaccinated or not, one is not truly free, because one still is being told that it is necessary to wear a facemask, practice social distancing, and to avoid taking unnecessary risks being around other people.

Of the various pharma and biotech companies at large on the COVID-19 scene, Pfizer is one of the most commonly used. It is an interesting fact to note that in 2017, the agency received a warning for having contaminants such as cardboard and glass discovered inside vials. FDA spoke of the agency and claimed,

"it posed a severe risk of harm to patients and indicated that the facility's process for manufacturing sterile injectable products was out of control."

Both Moderna and Pfizer have thousands of reported cases of patients having experienced side effects varying from little too severe. Most of these cases of adverse reactions occur only when patients receive the second dose of the experimental vaccine. Dr. Robert Wachter, chief of medicine at UCSF says,

"side effects after the second shot are more common because the immune response to the second shot is even stronger than the response to the first shot."

In the U.S. military, they line members up and usher them through a hallway where about a dozen or more fellow military members on staff, stand waiting to administer various shots as members walk through like an assembly line. It is mandatory for all active-duty members to receive whatever vaccines or shots the U.S. government may deem necessary. Unfortunately, this is never a low number of shots and in the event of a deployment, can result in receiving so many, that one is left with an angry, putrid, painful, pustule that eventually becomes a scar. I will confess that every single time that I received a shot in this fashion or for the influenza, I fell horribly ill for up to three weeks at a time. These are not the kinds of side effects that are even worth mentioning and are not the ones that people who oppose the use of COVID-19 experimental vaccines, are complaining about or becoming terrified of. The side-effects of these experimental vaccines that also cause me to fear the future like never before, is the kinds that go undetected and untested for, because of the nature of its severity and as a result of the accelerating the release and dispensing of experimental vaccines. Scientific and medical experts decades ago, calculated these durations for each phase in accordance with proven efficacy and results. These measures allowed for the necessary time that it takes to detect some of the more serious long-term side effects or interactions. For the CDC and EMA to ignore decades of evidence proving that the safety and effectiveness of trial vaccines increase when manufacturers and government agencies adhere to the meticulous and methodical process of development and testing that is set in place. It is not surprising at all that these four experimental vaccines are meeting controversy.

Proven by Dr. Tenpenny, the pharmaceutical industry has been trying to produce a vaccine for the coronavirus for years and was never approved because they were never able to get the trials to verify it was safe for human testing. Even for the vaccines for COVID-19, complete clinical trials were later bypassed only because of the Emergency Utilization of Authorization and the world pandemic status. If you conduct a little research on the results from the animal trials that had previously been rejected by FDA, CDC, and the EMA, you will learn that this was due to a failure to produce evidence of effectuality and safety. During these trials, animals that were tested whether they had been injected with the coronavirus at the start of the trial or not, both the experimental and the constant

HOW A SINGLE VIRUS BROUGHT HUMANITY TO ITS KNEES

subjects not only became infected or reinfected, but eventually grew extremely ill and died. It is alarming with a proven mortality rate of close to 0%, that over 150 pharmaceutical or biotech companies are currently developing versions of their own experimental vaccine. Dr. Tenpenny is just one example of someone who is more than qualified to speak truth about the COVID-19 vaccines and the threat they pose to humanity. Dr. Tenpenny served in a level 2 trauma center for twelve years, is emergency medical board certified, an osteopathic physician, and has spent more than 40,000 hours researching the use of vaccines and their effects on the human body and has been studying this research for the last twenty years. It is for this reason, I am going to reference her own research to give you a better understanding of what these experimental viruses are made of what they are intended to accomplish, and how they will irreversibly and negatively affect the human body.

 In high school science class, I had once conducted a simple but riveting experiment which involved a plastic bottle of soda and a pack of mentos. For anyone who has never seen what happens when these two substances react, give it a try one day, and the excitement will blow your cap off! When it comes to mentioning volatile materials that must be kept stable by controlled temperatures or pressure, the mind immediately rushes to thoughts of danger. And rightfully so. If the mass media, social media, or government is the only source that you receive information about COVID-19, this next fact will surely blow your mind. To get a sample of the Pfizer vaccine to remain stable, it must be stored at temperatures that are colder than the north pole otherwise, it will not hold together. When these samples of trial vaccine are being transported from a lab, into solution, and finally injected into your arm, it is kept under this controlled condition. No such extremes were ever required for the transport of a vaccine meant for human distribution. Both Moderna and Pfizer use mRNA messaging meant to spark the production of an anti-spike protein antibody. To mention it again, all of the pharma community's past attempts to construct such a vaccine for coronaviruses failed because it was deemed unsafe. Please do not allow mass media to deceive you into believing things have suddenly changed…they are still as unsafe if not more unsafe, now than they were prior. All four of the existing trial vaccines are totally experimental. Stating otherwise, would be a grand leap from the truth and if stated by a physician or a scientist in the field, it would cause legal commotion without the protection of the EUA. Another fact worth mentioning is that if it were not for the EUA, all four vaccines would have been unauthorized and otherwise deemed unsafe by FDA and EMA. **Nothing has changed about how unsafe these trial vaccines are**.

Strictly for educational purposes, I will share what was learned from studying and reviewing from Dr. Tenpenny. Back at the lab, Pfizer and Moderna inject small pieces of genetic material (this is a process that has never been done before in the history of medicine and never tested for its long-term safety) into synthetic or manmade mRNA. This mRNA consists of an encoded message for a specific type of protein. This process can be compared to delivering an envelope telling someone to search for a particular person you are wanting to find. Once the message from mRNA has been released, this encoded message is then sent to your own cellular DNA and finally back out into your cells. The objective and scientific idea behind this process, is to create antibodies to bind with this spike-protein. To make a protein called spike protein, which are extremely unstable, the sample invites itself into the ribosomes which control the manufacturing of proteins in the body. This process occurs naturally to repair an injury or attend to a cellular need, however, in the case of these two trial vaccines, this is an induced and synthetic process. Technicians at Pfizer and Moderna inject the genetic material created in the lab inside of a lipid coating made of some other materials that have never been used before or tested. Ultimately proving again, that there has not been the amount of research and testing needed to evaluate these vaccines for safety. One particular material that is used to make up the exterior coating of these samples, is called polyethylene glycol, which is known to cause big allergic reactions in humans. If one of the constituents used in this lipid coating is known to be toxic, how many others could be as well? If you are someone who has received one of these trial vaccines, the anti-spike antibody, that is meant to be there to keep your body from getting sick, can have direct adverse effects on tissues such as liver, heart, lungs, or kidney, if these populate incorrectly. Ironically, causing you to become sick and even making it possible for you to become infected with COVID-19 virus again. A fact that makes sense and is supported by the reported number of vaccinated people who have tested positive post-vaccination and for a second time. If this already does not sound horrendous enough, the synthetic Pfizer or Moderna introduced Anti-antibody can become combined to your DNA cells and irreversibly change them by way of a process called transfection. When this process occurs, foreign nucleic acids are introduced into cells to produce **genetically modified cells.** The proof is in the pudding. This scientific study is known as, analytical, and bioanalytical chemistry, and it is exactly what was aforementioned as having never been approved when applied to gene therapy and vaccines for coronaviruses, because it has always proven to be unsafe. According to the National Center for Biotechnology Information,

"Transfection is a powerful analytical tool for study of gene function and regulation and protein function."

What does all of that mean to you if you have already taken these experimental vaccines? It means you have participated in an unapproved and improperly tested experiment for gene therapy and that any adverse conditions are irreversible due to the fact, your cellular DNA is being involved in an unnatural cellular exchange (Tenpenny, Sherri, American Physician, 2021). Among these long-term negative effects, Dr. Tenpenny mentions, autoimmune disease, cardiovascular conditions, and neurological conditions. She claims,

"Some people are going to die from the vaccine directly. But a large number of people are going to start getting horribly sick and get all kinds of autoimmune diseases."

In a terrifying contrast to these facts you have now learned, President Joe Biden says,

"The U.S. will have enough coronavirus vaccines for all adults by the end of May."

It amazes me how politicians, WHO, CDC, EMA, leaders, and mass media, can push and in some places, force, entire populations of people to partake in an experiment by pharmaceutical and biotech companies like Pfizer or Moderna, who were only able to push these experimental products forward because of the pandemic status and EUA. It is also wrong and against human rights, for the government to be interfering the way that it is worldwide, censoring every physician, politician, or scientist, who blows the whistles or even simply states facts that contradict or disprove their own claims of validity, efficacy, intention, and concerns for safety.

In April 2021, the most credible possible voice spoke out against the use of these trial vaccines. Geert Vanden Bossche, DVM, PhD, is an independent and highly acclaimed virologist and vaccine expert who tirelessly worked alongside the Global Alliance of Vaccine and Immunization (GAVI) during the Ebola epidemic and served as the Senior Program Officer at the Bill & Melinda Gates Foundation, where he led the research and development of most of the world's vaccines. After being asked why mass vaccination campaigns are promoting dominance of selective immune escape variants, Dr. Bossche, responds,

"I repeat with utmost urgency my call for a public scientific debate with the WHO, qualified experts and authorities worldwide."

The man is challenging the entire WHO on its decision to not only mass vaccinate, but to carelessly force and pressure the world into taking these experimental drugs. Dr. Bossche is a highly passionate vaccine guy who holds no criticism on the use of vaccines but encourages people to

"use the right vaccine at the right place and don't use it in the heat of a pandemic on millions and millions of people."

He then goes on to express his grave and dire concerns,

HOW A SINGLE VIRUS BROUGHT HUMANITY TO ITS KNEES

"We are going to pay a huge price for this. And I am becoming emotional because I am thinking of my children, of the younger generation; it is just impossible what we are doing. We do not understand the pandemic. We have been turning it into an artificial pandemic. Who can explain where all these highly infectious variants come from? I can explain it. We have not seen this in previous pandemics. Because in **natural pandemics**, every single time, there was the immunity was low enough so that the virus did not need to escape. What we are now doing is merely chasing this virus and it becomes increasingly infectious and this is just a situation that is completely out of control."

Deeming the situation, a massive public health emergency, he explains that the science proves that mass infection prevention and mass vaccination with experimental COVID-19 vaccines in the midst of the pandemic can only breed highly infectious variants. This science is aligned with what was forementioned about the cellular manipulation and synthesis that is occurring in the human bodies of all people who are receiving the trial vaccines for COVID-19. However, what his expertise in virology and vaccines explains further, is how this synthetically induced manipulation will affect the immune system in a way that will completely destroy it. As the world discovers the abounding non-lethality of the COVID-19 virus, it will soon experience something far incredibly worse as a result of taking these experimental vaccines. In Dr. Bossche's own words,

"The fact is, there are long-lived anti-bodies (spike-proteins created as a result of trial vaccines) which have high specificity of course, for the virus, they outcompete our natural antibodies. Because natural antibodies have a very broad spectrum, but they have low affinity, the specific antibody (synthetic antibody created with COVID-19 trial vaccines) will still continue to outcompete your natural antibody. And that is a huge problem because these natural antibodies, they provide you with broad protection. This protection is very variant-unspecific. It does not matter which variant you get; it doesn't even matter what type of coronavirus you get; they will protect you. Unless of course, you depress this level of innate immunity (natural synthesis and functionality of antibodies in a human immune system) or if it is, for example, out competed by long-lived specific antibodies (synthetic antibodies synthesized by COVID-19 trial vaccines. And so, it is not like you missed it, ok let us try again. No! You did some harm. This is different from the rest. Immunizing somebody is installing a new software on your computer. These antibodies will be recalled every single time you are encountering a coronavirus. You cannot just erase this. So, this is very serious."

What this science is explaining is that by taking these trial vaccines, you are literally destroying your innate immune system antibodies that were nonspecific and could have handled any of the coronavirus variants. Our natural immune systems are designed to accomplish exactly this. By being vaccinated by COVID-19 experimental vaccines, you assure yourself that there will be no natural antibodies inside of you to fight the variant coronaviruses or other sicknesses Because the spike-protein antibodies created by these trial vaccines are specifically created to only attack and defend against the original SARS-CoV-2 virus, they will completely compromise the natural antibodies which are broadly unspecific and designed to attack and defend the body against any sickness, putting anyone who has received these trial vaccines in serious danger of infection from any variant of the coronavirus or some other sickness such as pneumonia. Dr. Bossche continues,

"It is a global problem we are talking about. It is not an individual adverse event. **It is a global problem of making this virus increasingly infectious because we leave it all the time, the chance and opportunity to escape an immune system and drive it up to a level where the virus is so infectious that we can no longer control it.**"

Before the mass vaccinations, humanity by the grace and perfection of its natural immunity systems, would have greatly prevailed against this pandemic as it has prevailed every time in the past. However, after this mass vaccination from leaky trial vaccines that manipulate and compromise the natural immune systems, humanity awaits in the palms of the reaper and is completely susceptible to a real mass pandemic far greater than the threat we could have or would have ever encountered to begin with. These experimental COVID-19 vaccines are increasing the strength and infectiousness of the coronavirus and in turn, creating variants that have begun to attack and affect populations of youth and healthy groups that otherwise, were unaffected by the SARS-CoV-2 original virus. A virus requires a living host to survive. By definition, all living organisms strive to survive and remain alive. The coronavirus does not benefit if its host perishes which is why over time, it gradually weakens itself so that it can remain and spread through more hosts without actually killing the hosts and itself. This is nature and how our natural immune systems manage to prevail and prevail again over various sickness. As the virus weakens itself for survival, our natural immunity systems remain intact and in a healthy body, grow stronger in its natural ability to defend against sicknesses.

On his coverage of Dr. Bossche's interview, Del Bigtree of *Highwire*, told viewers,

"These COVID-19 trial vaccines are turning hundreds of millions and millions of people around the world into a gigantic gain-of-function laboratory."

This situation is not involving a natural virus and our general response with these trial vaccines, has caused the birth of an unnatural pandemic whereas, the original was an underperforming virus. With most of the world's leader's moving towards mandates where people are forced to become vaccinated whether they wish to or not, because proof of vaccination is being required to work, travel, or function in society, this problem is growing larger and larger on a global scale. Dr. Bossche confesses to anyone who has taken or is planning to take the trial vaccines,

"You are at the same time, losing the most precious part of your immune system that you could ever imagine of, and that is your innate immune system. Because innate antibodies, natural antibodies, the circulatory IgMs, will be out competed by this antigen specific antibodies binding to the virus. It is a long-lived suppression, and you lose. Every protection against any viral variant or coronavirus variant etcetera. So, this means you are left with just no signal immune response; its numb, your immune system has become null; it is all done.

The antibodies won't work anymore and your innate immunity has been completely bypassed. And this is while highly infectious variants are circulating. And people, please read what I have posted because it is pure science."

Not only have I included sources from Dr. Bossche's research and webpage, but I will also share his more scientific explanation of what is occurring in people's bodies as a result of receiving these various COVID-19 experimental vaccines,

"First, in order for more emerging more infectious variants to enhance their potency and become well established, they must adapt to the suboptimal immune pressure they escaped from. To adapt viruses to grow at high infectious titers under suboptimal conditions, it is critical to passage the virus repeatedly under the same 'stress' conditions. Likewise, repeated person-to-person transmission of a highly mutable virus under similarly selective, suboptimal immune pressure would enable 'training' of selected immune escape variants. This will ultimately result in an adaptation of the viral variant and thereby enable full-fledged replication under conditions which initially restricted its replication. All more infectious Sars-CoV-2 are characterized by mutations that are directed at spike (S) protein (herein called S variants'). Selection of S-directed mutations enables enhanced binding of these variants to the ACE-2 cell receptor. By virtue of their enhanced binding to cell receptors on respiratory epithelial cells, variants are able to overcome limitations in infectiousness imposed by S-specific antibodies (Abs). In the absence of infection prevention measures or mass vaccination campaigns, spontaneously occurring S variants have no opportunity to compete with circulating wild virus as there is no selective immune pressure mechanism promoting their adaptation to the human host. Lastly, those who are in the process of seroconverting as a result of Coronavirus infection will not be susceptible to re-infection by another CoV due to antiviral innate immunity (natural immunity response / no CoV trial vaccine). In cases of mass vaccination however, there is plenty of opportunity for spontaneously occurring S variants to experience selective immune pressure. Mass vaccination campaigns will cause large, not previously primed cohorts of the population to seroconvert against S protein and to even maintain suboptimal Abs for quite some time. (eg. In those waiting for the second dose of a 2-shot vaccine) while being exposed to spontaneously emerging viral variants. Such cohorts include people who have not previously been infected at all as well as subjects who have been asymptomatically infected and only exhibited short-lived Ab titers, presumably due to lack of adequate priming. Mass vaccination of vulnerable groups does not abrupt viral transmission chains but increasingly redirects transmission events to asymptomatic carriers (vaccinated subjects as well as not yet vaccinated young and healthy people, several of whom experienced asymptomatic infection without mounting long-lived Ab titers). As ongoing mass vaccination campaigns are shifting the 'reservoir' of viral transmission to asymptomatically infected subjects (whether vaccinated or not), the likelihood for unvaccinated, previously asymptomatically infected subjects to experience re-infection with Sars-Cov-2 while being endowed with suboptimal and short-lived anti-S Abs substantially increases. As mass vaccination campaigns have started in the vulnerable population, not only vaccinated subjects, but also no yet vaccinated younger age groups will become a breeding ground for new infectious variants."

The rarest and most praised art in the world, is protected from tainting or blemishing by museums and private owners. What makes a masterpiece a masterpiece, is its authenticity; the human immunity systems are biological masterpieces. Like a prized painting or an ancient relic, these immunity systems must be protected from tainting and blemishing. Dr. Bossche is emphasizing this point when he scientifically explains how these very inauthentic anti-bodies are destroying what was already a perfect masterpiece inside the human body. Insidiously, the elite scientists and government leaders who are behind these experimental vaccines remain silent and idle in their golden shadows while selfless and courageous men and women like Dr. Bossche, fight against the misinformation in an attempt to share the truth. A truth that could save millions and millions of lives. Unfortunately, in midst of even a global crisis, corruption and avarice are proving to prevail. It is increasingly difficult for these individuals of moral courage to properly inform the populace of the facts because the WHO,

CDC, and most world leaders, are censoring, blocking, or even mislabeling, everything that they attempt to share mainstream.

During my research, I listened to Tony Robbins interview top physicians and epidemiologist and infectious disease experts who had videos of them sharing statistics such as the number of actual patients at the emergency room during the outbreak, taken down on social media platforms and in articles. For every article or message of truth that is shared by an expert or a physician, another article appears trying to disclaim the facts or demean the professional who is only trying to inform the public of the truth and what needs to be heard to truly stay safe. It is easy for these leaders and mass media to distort the truth in an attempt to keep up and defend the lies. All this declaring that these experimental vaccines are not experimental and claiming that they have underwent scrutinous testing to prove their effectiveness and safety, can be easily silenced by pointing out the fact that simply because they went and altered the fine print, changed the rules mid-game, does not magically rise reality to actually make the trial vaccines effective and safe. Simply because a voice qualified to speak on the COVID-19 matter speaks against what is being produced on the mainstream, does not make that voice any less qualified nor does it make it a voice of a conspiracist. They are stripping people of their constitutional rights to speak. Every person has a right to express their opinions. Facts do not lie…people lie.

It is equally insidious when the WHO and these experimental vaccine creators selectively withhold information. According to Dr. Tenpenny, Johnson & Johnson use a hollowed-out adenovirus that they fill with a premade genetic and synthetic material. Within the material, PCR.C6 tissue (human embryonic retinal cells) from previously aborted fetuses and HEK (human embryonic kidney cells) which is also from previously aborted fetuses, can be found. Not informing the general public of its use of an extremely controversial tissue, is an injustice of and in itself. Of the population of women who have chosen to receive this vaccine, how many were feminist or anti-abortionist? The deception surrounding the COVID-19 pandemic is the real death-star.

HOW A SINGLE VIRUS BROUGHT HUMANITY TO ITS KNEES

Interestingly enough, there is evidence to suggest that this entire *Plandemic* had been part of a covert and sadistic agenda that had first been developed decades ago. Before she had been blackmailed by big Pharma and gagged by the U.S. government, Judy Mikovits, PhD, was a widely respected member of the medical and scientific community. She is most well-known for her part in the research that helped create a way to manage HIV-AIDS and for her twenty-years of work alongside Dr. Frank Ruscetti, one of the founding fathers of human retrovirology. In one of her most recent publications called *Plague of Corruption,* with former attorney Kent Heckenlively, JD, Robert F. Kennedy Jr. proffers the following words in his foreword to this work,

"This account by Judy Mikovits and Kent Heckenlively is vitally important both to the health of our children and the vitality of our democracy. My father believed moral courage to be the rarest species of bravery. Rarer even than the physical courage of soldiers in battle or great intelligence. He thought it the one vital quality required to salvage the world. If we are to continue to enjoy democracy and protect our children from the forces that seek to commoditize humanity, then we need courageous scientists like Judy Mikovitz who are willing to speak truth to power, even at terrible personal cost."

Is it by mere coincidence, that all of the major and even minor voices of moral courage acting against the COVID-19 lies, are being censored and silenced? When millions of people are storming the streets around the world and demanding the truth be spoken, I think it is prudent to believe that it is not. Dr. Anthony Fauci and Bill Gates are the two most suspicious and shady faces at the forefront of the COVID-19 predicament. Dr. Fauci seems to have always found his way into the clutches of conspiracy theorist. As I like to say, the woodpecker only pecks the steel pole once before it moves over to the tree and pecks a hole with natural ease. If Dr. Fauci, chief of the National Institute of Allergy and Infectious Diseases (NIAID), was not committing wrongs, then he would not continuously find his way at the top of the list for most publicly mistrusted health officials from then until now. In 1983, Dr. Fauci along with Big Pharma and Dr. Redwood of CDC, was discovered to have been the reason why the conformation and release of valuable research on HIV-AIDS was unnecessarily paused. Thousands stormed the NIH campus in protest of the ways Dr. Fauci was mishandling the research situation. Truth be told, he and Dr. Redwood had financial interest in the patent for pharmaceutical solutions being developed at this time which alludes to a major conflict of interest and very well could have been the reason why they had delayed the release to the community suffering from HIV-AIDS. As forementioned in this book, he has not done much better at handling the COVID-19 pandemic. While America and the World eagerly waited to hear him speak on the virus, it seemed he had become more like a pawn against the Trump administration. At the very least, mass media certainly made it appear so. Even after the close of the election, it had been discovered that Dr. Fauci had made over twenty different false statements about COVID-19, the vaccines, and the effectiveness of the draconian methods. It was also discovered that much of the funding given to the pharmaceutical giants for the development of these trial vaccines for COVID-19, came from no other than, Bill Gates. To make this process even more shady, by way of the Bayh-Dole Act, a regulation that impacts the ownership of patent rights on intellectual property, Gates, an individual with no expertise or qualifications in vaccines or medicine, was authorized to heavily influence the research and development behind the four vaccines that are being forced upon the world populace. Like Dr. Fauci had a conflict of interest with Pharma and the development of drugs for HIV-AIDS, Gates, and his unqualified and bias influences on the COVID-19 vaccines, presents a major conflict of interest and a lack of assiduity. When the WHO receives nearly all of its funding from the Gates Foundation, it is even more reasonable to assume the claims made out against him, Dr. Fauci, and the WHO. If he is the one that provides the funding that is required for the WHO and these vaccine manufacturers to operate, not doing what he, a nonexpert, says, could potentially lead to a damming of that funding. There is incontestable evidence that Gates has too powerful an influence on WHO, the vaccine developers, and world government, concerning the COVID-19 pandemic. Gates says,

HOW A SINGLE VIRUS BROUGHT HUMANITY TO ITS KNEES

"Normalcy only returns when we've largely vaccinated the entire global population."

This idea has proved to stand true in only a few specific cases. Vaccination is a controversial science. However, the world's population continues to rapidly increase despite the fact that the majority of the world rarely receives a single one. This brings Gates's theory to an intellectual trial. Is vaccination for everyone really necessary? During a conference, he discussed he and his team's plan for accomplishing mass vaccination using gene editing. In this process, natural cells in the body's DNA are synthetically modified. Sound familiar? This is the same science that the mRNA trial vaccines for COVID-19 are using. Quoting Gates himself,

"Another new approach that the Foundation is very enthused about is the ORGAN-ON-A-CHIP. An in simple terms, the technology allows invitro modeling of human organisms in a way that mimics how they work in the human body. There is some degree of simplification. Most of these systems are single organ systems, they do not repopulate everything. But some of the key elements we do see there, including some of the disease state. For example, with the liver, the intestines, and the kidneys. It lets us understand drug kinetics. We also are culturing a human intestine and testing microbiome upon it that will let us understand the interactions between microbiome nutrients and pathogens in a systematic way. Another area that looks to have promise is, the vaginal microbiome. It is pretty clear that an imbalance there dramatically increases the risk of HIV acquisition and because that is very prevalent in Africa, that is the explanation as to why the disease spreads in larger numbers there and less so than other locations. So, the question is then, can you intervene in a way that changes that risk. Another organ-on-a-chip that's very promising for us is the lymphoid **organoids to understand vaccine responses that could let us develop vaccines faster and understand things like adjuvants that are very critical for a lot of the new vaccines that we are working on.**"

Judy Mikovits confirms that there are no vaccines currently on schedule from any RNA virus that work. This fact can also be validated by the records of all previous trials on WHO or EMA webpages and by government records of approved vaccine products. It is also a fact, that these theories constituting the use of nanotechnology to induce cellular replication and tracing, have yet to be properly tested and approved. What does this tell us about the COVID-19 trial vaccines? It further confirms what we already know to be true: they are one hundred percent experimental and have never proven successful in either tests for human safety or for effectivity at preventing a subject from becoming infected or reinfected. It also proves that the WHO is so heavily influenced by the Gates Foundation, that it has adopted Gate's suggestion to practice gene therapy on the entire world. It does not matter to Gates or to any of the pharma companies if millions of people lose their lives and billions are negatively afflicted. They all stand to make hundreds of billions from the worldwide distribution of the experimental vaccines for COVID-19. Whereas the medical professionals and scientific experts that are stepping up and speaking against these types of gene manipulating drugs, care so deeply about the public's safety, that they are losing their jobs and suffering their reputation to do so.

During his 2010 TED talk, Gates shared with the audience and viewers,

"Let us see which one of these numbers needs to get down to zero; **probably one of these numbers is probably going to need to get pretty near to zero.** (Eq. ref. TED, 2020. CO_2=P [People] x S [Services per person] x E [Energy per service] x C [CO_2 per unit energy]) First we have got population. The world today has 6.8 billion people and that is headed up to about nine billion. Now, **if we do a really great job on new vaccines**, health care, reproductive services, **we could lower that by perhaps ten or fifteen percent**."

More than ten years before the outbreak of COVID-19, Bill Gates told the world that part of his plan for reducing the world's production of CO_2, is **using vaccines, health care, and reproductive services.** He also stated that by doing so, **we**

could eliminate ten to fifteen percent of the population which equals about one billion twenty million people!

During a different TED talk in March 2015, he told audiences,

"If anything kills over ten million people in the next few decades, it's most likely to be a virus rather than a war. Not missiles, but microbes. We are not ready for the next epidemic. With EBOLA, the problem was not that we had a system that didn't work well enough, the problem was we didn't have a system at all. So, next time, we might not be so lucky. You can have a virus where people feel well enough while they are infectious, that they get on a plane or they go to a market. The source of the virus could be a natural epidemic like EBOLA or it could be **bioterrorism**. And so, there are things, that would literally make things a thousand times worse. **Let's look at a model of a virus that is spread through the air like the Spanish flu** back in 1918. **It would spread throughout the world very, very, quickly. About thirty million people die from this pandemic.** So, this is a serious problem, and we should be concerned. But in fact, we can build a really good response system. We have the benefit of all the science and technology that we talk about here. **We got cell phones to get information from the public and to get information out to them. We have satellite maps where we can see where people are, and we can see where they're moving. We have advances in biology that should dramatically change the turn-around time to look at a pathogen and be able to make drugs and vaccines that fit for that pathogen."**

These are two instances where Gates has eerily described an environment almost exactly as that of the COVID-19 era. What makes this even more sadistic, is he stated these notions five and ten years prior. In his second TED talk, he even mentions things such as, bioterrorism, comparisons to an airborne virus and to the Spanish Flu, government dissemination of information via media, control and restrictions on movement, and advances in biology that could **accelerate the rate of which vaccines are developed and released.** All of the preceding points are points that have proven true with COVID-19 and the trial vaccines today. Before the end of the talk, Gates continues,

"NATO has a mobile unit that can deploy very rapidly. NATO does a lot of war games to check if people are well trained, do they understand about logistics, and the same radio frequency, so they are absolutely ready to go. So, those are the kinds of things that we need, to deal with an epidemic. So, what are the pieces? We need strong health care systems in poor countries. We need a medical reserve core. And then we need to pair those medical people with the military. **We need to do simulations. Germ games, not war games. To find out where the holes are.** The last time a germ game was done in the United States was back in 2001 and it didn't go so well. So far, the score is germs one people zero. Finally, **we need lots of advanced R&D in areas of vaccines and diagnostics. There are some big breakthroughs like the adeno associated virus that could work very, very, quickly**. Now, I don't have an exact budget for what this would cost but I'm quite sure it's very modest compared to the potential harm. **The world estimates that if we have a worldwide pandemic, global wealth will go down by over three trillion dollars and we would have millions and millions of deaths.**"

Gates urged world leaders, WHO, and world scientists, to create germ games and pandemic simulations. He referenced the use of adenoviruses in vaccines which is a primary component in the production of the Johnson & Johnson mRNA trial vaccine. And lastly, he predicted, or rather, he **forewarned**, the world of major losses to economy and lives. I'm sure as a child, many of you that are reading this, have enjoyed connecting the dots to form a picture in a children's book. Remember how easy that was? It is just as easy to connect the dots to form the whole picture of this COVID-19 *Plandemic*. Between Dr. Fauci, the WHO's, CDC's, EMA's and many world leader's, complete and obscene naivety, and ignorance of the sinister corruption afoot, and Bill Gates and his insidious plan of world depopulation, biosynthetic tracking, and gene therapy, there is no time for people to remain idle or blindly compliant. It is more likely, that the groups and peoples generously prelabeled as being naïve and ignorant, are in fact also in cahoots with Gates. Equally as important to mention, is the justifications for the rapid release of unapproved and improperly tested or researched trial vaccines.

Preventing the hospitals from being overwhelmed "again," became the underlying reason being used to justify the emergency utilization of experimental and unapproved vaccines. How do you explain the innumerous claims from around the planet about empty hospitals and secrets? A video of hospital staff in Brazil was circulating and depicted a nurse walking around pulling curtains to reveal empty beds and unused ventilators that were supposed to be filled with patients according to world media and WHO. In a conversation with Tony Robbins and 7 physicians and scientist, an account was shared about a hospital in California only having 4 COVID-19 patients while mass media was leading the world to believe the hospital was overwhelmed by patients with the virus. Any claims made about experiencing an adverse effect from taking the vaccines, are being belittled and downplayed. Hundreds of women have come forward expressing concern about how their menstrual flow and symptoms have become irregular and more severe only after having received the trial vaccines. One woman has experiencing bleeding for twenty days straight after having received the trial vaccine. Other reports indicate that reception of the vaccine caused an increase in the number of miscarriages. When the WHO, CDC, EMA, and mass media attempt to silver-tongue and downplay all of these claims, it is infuriating. None of these companies that provided the trial vaccines even went through proper and full procedures and so they therefore cannot accurately inform patients on whether the vaccine could potentially have adverse effects on menstrual cycles or pregnancy. The truth and fact are, they do not know what long-term effects will occur. But you should know based on what I have shared with you, that almost everything that Bill Gates had prescribed to the world back in 2015 about the next pandemic, has come true.

Some people may consider this and still be fine with assuming the risk. Others will only take the vaccines to avoid inconveniences, to keep jobs, or because of government mandating. At the end of the day, no matter the world situation, a person should be entitled to make decisions about their health. If I do not want to take an experimental vaccine but my brother does, we are both in the right because we both freely choose. The major problem arises from these companies not being able to fully inform people about these drugs which would have helped alleviate a majority of adverse effects and reports. Another major problem is with governments abusing citizen rights about their health by ordering them to take one of the trial vaccines, by creating the need for a vax passport that would greatly restrict the lives of citizens who do not wish to comply, and by treating those who choose to not get the vaccine with negative prejudice.

According to VAERS, the largest collection of adverse reports from vaccines, by April 2021, there are almost 30,000 adverse events to vaccines and almost 2,000 deaths in the U.S. alone. In the beginning of February 2021, CDC had reported 996 deaths to vaccines and from the last week in February to the first week in March, the number had risen from 1097 to 1278 deaths. Knowing that only about 10% of adverse events are said to be reported, so statistically, there could be nearly 50,000 adverse events or as many as 15,000 deaths from vaccines that are not being reported or properly reflected in reports of trial vaccine safety. At this rate, the increase in the number of adverse cases and deaths due to the experimental vaccines, will be drastic and devastating. It may also come as surprise to those who are "Pro-COVID-19 regime" that, the Pfizer ex-officio told the world not to reproduce after vaccination. What other reason other than they have no idea what possible interactions or adverse situations wither short or long-term, their experimental drug may cause. Here are the most current list of deaths and adverse reactions separated by trial vaccine from the European Database of Adverse Reactions of COVID-19 'vaccines'(EudraVigiliance):

BioTech Pfizer Experimental mRNA Vaccine Tozinameran (code BNT16262)	
Deaths: 3,760	**Adverse Injuries: 134,606**

Moderna mRNA Vaccine MRNA-1273 (RX-024417)	
Deaths: 1,801	Adverse Injuries: 13,426

JANSSEN (AD26.COV2.5) from Johnson & Johnson (Not readily available in EU – Lower Number of People Taken in Poll)	
Deaths: 15	Adverse Injuries: 170

Based on these reports, there is strong evidence of adverse effects from the COVID-19 trial vaccines and so people who desire to refrain from taking that risk, should be free to do so and not discriminated against in any of the ways that are being seen all around the world.

Pressure for adults to become vaccinated had only just begun to pick up in 2015. Not too many years prior to that year, there had been a huge push for children to receive vaccinations. Before these mass vaccinations, people still managed to maintain around the same life expectancy that is seen today. The human immunity systems are incredibly powerful tools against disease, viruses, and infections and they accomplish this without the need of manmade vaccinations. It is for this reason, up until December 2020, that people would never dream of leaders making a vaccination a mandatory requirement to travel or to work or pressuring the total populations into receiving the trial vaccines. And especially not a vaccine that is still experimental and that was created for a virus that effects less than 1% of the population. Having the freedom to decide on your own is a part of life and a part of what makes humanity able to prevail. If you accept the experimental vaccinations as even many members of my own family have, that was a decision that you made for yourself and for your own body. Don't cast judgement or act prejudice on those of us who also make a decision for ourselves but one that is not the same as your own.

It is without a doubt that some of the most brilliant and proficient minds are behind the construction of these vaccines. Be that as it may, the term *mad scientist*, did not come about for no reason. If this group of elite scientists and government leaders had nothing to hide and wanted only what was best for the safety and health of the public, they would not be censoring, withholding, and manipulating information as they are. If the experimental vaccines were really safe, approved, and thoroughly tested, the world population would have been informed of possible side effects both short and long term. They would have also been informed of the nature and science behind the trial vaccines. Finally, if the experimental vaccines had truly been tested, approved, and deemed safe, evidence of the vaccines approval and complete results would be available. But none of that information was ever shared with the public because information like the possible long term adverse effects or evidence the gene therapy proved to be effective, does not even exist. Instead, a government issued EUA was the one and only reason that these experimental vaccines were accelerated and released. We the people deserve to know the truth and the whole truth. To conclude this chapter, I am including the final note in Dr. Bossche's letter to the WHO, scientific experts, authorities, and populations, around the world, urging for the immediate cessation of all mass vaccinations for COVID-19. With agony and urgency, Dr. Bossche writes,

"While there is no time to spare, I have not received any feedback thus far. Experts and politicians have remained silent while obviously still eager to talk about relaxing infection prevention rules and 'springtime freedom'. My statements are based on nothing else but science. They should only be contradicted by science. While one can barely make any incorrect scientific statements without being criticized by peers, it seems like the elite of scientists who are currently advising our world leaders prefer to stay silent. Sufficient scientific evidence has been brought to the table. Unfortunately, it remains untouched by those who have the power to act. How long can one ignore the problem when there is at present massive evidence that viral immune escape is now threatening humanity? We can hardly say we did not know – or were not warned. In this agonizing letter I put all of my reputation and credibility at stake. I expect from you, guardians of mankind, at least the same. It is of utmost urgency. Do open the debate. By all means: turn the tide!"

Political Storms & Side Effects

"There's a difference between us. You think the people of this country exist to provide you with position. I think your position exists to provide those people with freedom. And I go to make sure that they have it."

William Wallace, *Braveheart*

World infamous genius, Albert Einstein, is credited with having once said, "Everybody is a genius. But if you judge a fish by its ability to climb a tree, it will live its whole life believing that it is stupid."

Before I even began to unzip and unpack this bag of facts and moot opinions, I was careful to include a content disclosure and a note to you, the reader. If you had originally decided to quickly turn and skip these pages, I implore you to revisit them. I especially encourage this if, as you are reading this, you are viewing the facts, ideas, and information presented, as only dancing projections of thought and bias from a man who is not professionally qualified to be speaking on a pandemic or a political conspiracy. Not once, have I claimed to be an expert epidemiologist or scientific source. Throughout its entirety, I have shared or based my ideas and information, on researched and sited fact and provided the most controversial of points via quotations from known individuals or parties within the pertaining fields. My mission is not to be a fish who seeks the approval of monkeys eager to judge me on my inability to climb a tree. Let it be known, I am a seeker of the truth and a sharer of the facts. My only wish is to be who I am; to be a fish who happily remains in the river because it is where it was made to be, where it can best function and thrive, and from where it can develop sound observations based on how life beneath the water is being affected by the actions or inactions of those who are outside of it. If you disagree with any of the ideas herein, hold to your disagreements. It is still a victory for me because ultimately, I am wanting to cause people to take a second look, a deeper glance, and a more earnest approach at the information mass media and government officials feed them. Further, please visit the litany of sources that can be referenced at the back of this book. If there is any information herein, that you have factual evidence to contest, I am a forever-student and a glass that is neither half empty nor half full, but one that is constantly eager to be filled-emptied-and filled again.

There is further question as to whether the SAR-COV-2 vaccine even exists or if it has somehow occurred naturally. According to scientist who study infectious disease, this family of viruses, were studied and manipulated in a laboratory where the animals were taken into the laboratory, bringing scientists to the ultimate reassurance, that this virus was not something that showed up at a wet market and suddenly transferred to humans. That process is known as accelerated viral evolution. It takes up to eight hundred years for a natural virus to occur and the COVID-19 virus, showed up in less than a decade, giving reasonable evidence it had been manipulated from SARS-COV-1 in a laboratory and later released. Based on official reports from CGTN, the U.S. government had provided a grant to the Wuhan lab and Institute of Virology, worth 3.7 million dollars and had continually funded its research of the transmission of the virus for the past decade. The Wuhan Virology Institute referred to the COVID-19 virus as a

"manmade coronavirus beyond human intelligence."

It is also a known fact that NIAD with Dr. Fauci at lead, had already been conducting experiments with the Wuhan lab in the past in regard to the coronavirus. This is one of the many instances when Dr. Fauci has neglected to admit facts to the public. Let it be known as well, that claims that Bill Gates has never funded the Virology and Infectious disease Laboratory in Wuhan, China, are gravely false. You can search directly on the Gates Foundation webpage and view the financial reports of all committed grants. Based on the financial reports depicted on this webpage, The Bill & Melinda Gates Foundation had funded the Wuhan lab and its coronavirus research and development for a total of forty-one months and in the total amount of $727,644. The Gates Foundation's financial commitments are shown to have first started in 2011 and continue through 2021. These figures and reports merely reflect known grants that were gifted to the Wuhan Lab, ground zero of the COVID-19 pandemic and allegedly, where the virus was created. Bear in mind, the Gates foundation generously supports "Global Development", a group that has funded millions worth to Wuhan and other virology labs worldwide to study coronaviruses and the development of vaccinations. I am not a person who believes in coincidences. Anyone who has an analytical mind, will not deny the irony in these findings. How is it, that the U.S. via Dr. Fauci and the NIH, and Bill Gates, via the Bill & Melinda Gates Foundation, were the primary sources of funding in the very lab where coronavirus research and development had been ongoing and where COVID-19 originated, and they are both the leading voices that have been dictating the current pandemic response? The four experimental vaccines were created using research and science from scientist and experts within the Gates Foundation that took place at its laboratories. It is even more ironic that the functions of the trial vaccines emulate what Gates had described during his TED talk years before. With only a little bit of research, I have gathered and presented overwhelming evidence that the COVID-19 pandemic is one-hundred percent political. From the outbreak in Wuhan to the EUA of experimental vaccines, this was a careful and insidious plan that had been developed decades ago. To use Gate's own words, is it a sinister "Germ Game" meant to accomplish his energy saving equation to drastically lessen the emission of CO_2 by way of depopulating the planet? One thing that we have learned for sure is that the government has crossed lines against the freedom of the people all around the world. The WHO, government leaders, and members of the elites, accumulated fear by using mass media like it was a growing and looming cloud of the black unknown. This cloud of fear then burst with torrential measures of restriction and abuse on civil liberties and rights. People were forced to remain indoors, seriously penalized for breaking these draconian laws, restricted from travel, forced to take a never-before-used and extremely invasive test, separated from loved ones, prohibited from work, required to wear masks that were not even provided at first, and then pressured or forced into receiving mass vaccination of experimental drugs that use never-before-used biotech. When you view the details and facts as a whole, the answer to the question of whether COVID-19 is a pandemic or a plandemic, becomes rather concrete.

It's all well and good for the WHO, government leaders, and mass media, to claim that they are doing what is in the public's best interest while keeping its safety at the top of its priorities, but a tree is known by its fruit. I will never forget the day that I was first introduced to that old idiom of wisdom that happens to derive from the synoptic gospel. A mentor and I had been discussing character and what that means when it comes to a young man, when he kindly told me that "a tree is known by its fruit and a man by his deeds". What type of fruit have these elite organizations and individuals that are in charge of making all the decisions during this heart-rending time, produced? Have you been enjoying the produce, or has it been making you as sick to stomach as it has been making me?

Tanzanian President, John Magufuli, is not only a brilliant mind who holds a PhD in chemistry, he is also an effective leader. Last summer, as the PCR tests were really being pushed by WHO, President Magufuli, conducted a little experiment where he used the PCR swabs on papaya and various animals before submitting them to the testing lab. To his surprise, these PCR tests had come back as being positive! In conclusion, President Magufuli spoke out to the world that the tests were producing false positive reports in order to make the actual number of positive cases seem higher than it really was. Whether this report is one hundred percent true is undetermined. However, based on the inordinate amount of evidence where the number of cases were being manipulated to reflect numbers that were far higher than what they actually were, I am more tempted to believe him over the WHO and elite scientists who combat the validity of his own declarations as well as those of countless physicians across the world. As I delve deeper into the politics and background of the PCR test, it is important to begin by reminding readers of the fact that this test has proven to provide varying results to include both false negatives and false positives, throughout the entire pandemic.

Trusting a test that measures substances qualitatively rather than quantitatively, and one that was originally created to be used as a scientific tool in a laboratory for the replication of DNA sequences and not as a diagnostic tool to detect viruses, seems unintelligible to say the least. The Bulgarian Pathology Association deems the use of COVID-19 PCR test as scientifically meaningless. These tests can be used to detect the genetic sequences of viruses but not the virus itself. To further support that the PCR method of testing is not scientifically sound or remotely accurate, the Bulgarian Pathology Association reminds the world via its webpage and based on its own research and that of labs throughout the world, there is no proof for the RNA being of viral origin. What does it mean if there is no proof of RNA originality or no evidence of the purified SARS-CoV-2 virus itself? This means that there is no scientific evidence to prove that the PCR tests accurately detect COVID-19 and that there are currently no existing samples of the isolated or purified virus. With no samples of the isolated SARS-CoV-2, there is no evidence of its existence period. All this time, the WHO, CDC, EMA, and world leaders, have been bullying the world in draconian-like fashion and instilling mass hysteria, because of the results from a test that is yet to be proven scientifically sound or even effective at detecting SARS-CoV-2. From the pathologists themselves,

"And because the PCR tests are calibrated for gene sequences (in this case RNA sequences because SARS-CoV-2 is believed to be an RNA virus), we have to know that these gene snippets are part of the looked-for-virus. And to know that, correct isolation and purification of the presumed virus has to be executed. Hence, we have asked the science teams, of relevant papers which are referred to in the context of SARS-CoV-2 for proof whether the electron-microscope shots depicted in their in vitro experiments show purified viruses. But not a single team could answer that question with 'yes' – and NB., nobody said purification was not a necessary step. We only got answers like 'No, we did not obtain an electron micrograph showing the degree of purification.'"

HOW A SINGLE VIRUS BROUGHT HUMANITY TO ITS KNEES

If the information from pathologists at BPA has not yet satisfied your thirst for evidence, perhaps a message from the inventor of the Polymerase Chain Reaction (PCR) himself, will suffice. Kary Mullis had invented the PCR test for gene sequencing and is quoted having stated that it was not effective at detecting free infectious viruses. Although, he did not directly mention SARS-CoV-2, you should get the point. Scientific evidence has provided incomprehensible evidence that the PCR tests were merely a tool used to further the reach of mass hysteria and manipulation as well as an egregious scientific overlook. However, the tests are still being forced upon the world populace and despite the invalidity of the results that the COVID-19 PCR tests yield, it brought humanity to its knees. Billions have lost jobs, billions are starving, billions are still restricted from traveling or from reuniting with loved ones, and billions are being deceived into accepting mass vaccination as an answer. The only reason why the world's leaders were so easily manipulated and pawned is because of the false reports of cases and deaths due to COVID-19. The CDC and FDA are quoted having warned the public on several different occasions that their test results may be either falsely negative or falsely positive. They even admitted the inconsistency yet still pushed the hysteria and false reports. Without these invalid results from the PCR tests, none of these insidious plans could have continued.

For the entirety of the COVID-19 pandemic, politics have always played the coocoo bird. There is an agenda and there always was an agenda. Just two years ago in 2019, the WHO warned the world that vaccination critics were among the top ten threats to global health. Subsequently, millions of people suddenly become leery of taking the COVID-19 trial vaccines. It almost seems like they had planned for this to happen. All across Europe, millions of people are flooding the streets to defend their freedoms and rights, to demand an end to the lockdowns, restrictions, and vaccinations. Many nations around the world have begun mandating vaccination and severely hindering the lives of anyone who opts out. In the United States military, DOD members are pressure and enticed to "immunize" by the issuance of benefits of travel, fitness, and leisure, that are not otherwise provided to those who opt to not be immunized. Further oppressing those who freely choose not to partake in mass vaccination of experimental vaccines, the U.S. government is restricting only unvaccinated individuals to adhere to previously enforced draconian mandates. This is a direct violation to a person's freedom of health and constitutional rights. As more and more specialists come forward to share the truth about the pandemic and the dangers of the trial vaccines, the number of nonvaccinated people increases. To battle this rise in resistance, many experts, and former mainstream journalists, such as John O'Sullivan, believe the government and WHO are furtively planning to use the PCR tests to vaccinate the unwilling. As ludicrous as this may come across, John Hopkins University has been tirelessly developing a way of accomplishing just that.

Miniature micro-devices called 'Theragrippers,' were developed to attach to the mucosa linings in the body and to then release a drug or toxin. Once these tiny devices gradually become released, they are passed through the gastrointestinal system. According to John Hopkin's University,

"Theragrippers are administer with a cotton swab. A theragripper is about the size of a speck of dust and each swab contains dozens of tiny devices."

Published results from animal trials were posted in *Science Advances* on October 28, 2020 and the article confirms that the technology proved to be effective:

"Here we report that GI parasite-inspired active mechanochemical therapeutic grabs, or theragrippers, can survive 24 hours in the gastrointestinal tract of live animals by autonomously adhering to mucosal tissue. We also observe a remarkable six-fold increase in elimination half-life when using ripper-mediated delivery of the model analgesic ketorolac tromethamine. These results provide excellent evidence that shape-shifting and self-locking microdevices improve the effectiveness of long-term drug delivery." (Science Advances, Oct. 2020)

If the potential use of this technology as a tool to unknowingly vaccinate the unvaccinated is not horrifying enough, SD Biosensor, Abbott, and Nadal, performed an analysis from November 2020 until March 2021, on PCR swab

HOW A SINGLE VIRUS BROUGHT HUMANITY TO ITS KNEES

samples in an undisclosed hospital laboratory in Bratislava, Slovakia, that potentially proves the elite's agenda is far more sinister and intentional than imaginable. By using microscopes, it was determined that (Defense Advanced Research Project Agency – developed by the United States Department of Defense for the development of emerging technologies for use by the military) **Darpa hydrogel and lithium were present within the hollow nylon fibers of the swabs**. Their findings showed that the saliva of a human who had overcame COVID-19 naturally and had antibodies, was disintegrated by the Darpa hydrogel crystal structures whereas when Ivermectin was applied, the Darpa Hydrogel Crystal structures were permanently gone. When Darpa Hydrogel was applied to blood cell samples, the blood cells were completely disintegrated. It also causes blood to clot within seconds which damages and clogs blood vessels. For anyone who has no idea what Darpa hydrogel or lithium is and to what degree of significance they may have over the human body,

"Darpa Hydrogel is an artificial substance that creates a converter between the electromagnetic signal and a living cell, tissue, or organ. Converts an electromagnetic signal from a transmitter to a signal which a living cell understands and responds to."

Lithium is an extremely toxic unnaturally occurring element in the body that negatively influences the pineal gland and in turn, manipulates one's ability to socially interact. What makes the presence of both of these substances on PCR swabs so terrifying is that when together, they completely destroy the pineal gland and essentially render a person into a biorobot that can be controlled via electromagnetic impulses or by frequencies such as 5G. These scientists also observed that mRNA significantly reduces the lifespan of a living organism based on past experimentation and results. They have also found that Darpa hydrogel hollow nylon fibers are being used in FFP2 class plastic respirators as well as the COVID-19 PCR swabs. As the PCR test is unnecessarily administered far into the nasal passageway, it only makes sense that it is an attempt to ensure traces of these substances enter the body in close proximity with the target pineal gland.

After being forced to take a PCR test in both nostrils eight separate times, I have experienced chronic headaches, congestion, fatigue, insomnia, altered mood, sporadic depression, and mesenteric adenitis which lasted more than two months with severe pain and swelling in various visceral organs. There were never conclusive results to what had caused that particular symptom, but it had only occurred after receiving a COVID-19 PCR test. This analysis of test sticks for COVID-19 provides evidence and confirmation of genocide. What is preventing a unanimous declaration of such an extensive accusation from being made is the refusal by government, WHO, and PCR manufacturers, to permit tests such as the one performed in Bratislava, worldwide. It is often easy to identify the culprit by pointing out which man or woman refuses to take his or her hands from out of his or her pockets.

Netflix aired a series called *Altered Carbon* where in this futuristic society, the human body is referred to as a "sleeve" and can be swapped in and out like attire by the elite class. A person's "soul or being" is compressed and stored into what is known as a "disc." Exactly like a computer's RAM and ROM, the disc is inserted in a sleeve of ones choosing. People are essentially patented by the governing force in this show and certain sleeves are militarized or synthetically adapted to perform specific functions. This series could not be anymore science fiction and yet, there is evidence to suggest that there is an elite group or force that is desiring to accomplish something eerily similar to what is depicted in this fictitious world.

There is no doubt that claiming the DNA manipulation that has been proven to be induced by these experimental mRNA vaccines can lead to one theorizing the possibility of people-patents. But after collecting copious amounts of evidence, one can be almost conclusive in stating that there is an elite agenda to accomplish exactly this. Bill Gates openly shared his hopes for quantum-dot and many nations are already in the process of pushing such an instrument that embeds into one's integumentary systems to perform and track a variety of things such as vaccination record or even GPS location. Government leaders are being manipulated by Gates and his group of elites who are claiming that this technology is simply to better monitor and control the spread of COVID-19. There is literally no telling what else this biotech device will be capable of accomplishing. It is being designed, developed, and manufactured, by the Gates Foundation who is then turning around and presenting it to world leaders. There is no need to embed an electronic device into a human body whether under the guise of simply storing medical data or tracking people's movements. It is reducing human beings to product and makes the argument about the government allowing people to be patented, seem more and more realistic and less and less science fiction. Former Federal Emergency Management Agency (FEMA) operative, Celeste Solum, believes that we are on the verge of having our biological self completely compromised. In a recent interview, she solemnly warned the world,

"Anyone who has taken a COVID test, they have placed a magnetic beacon; you have been tagged. You have been barcoded. And I'm going to provide you with that evidence."

From this interview and from some mining of my own, I have discovered some of the most horrifying facts such as the existence and scientific influence of an agency known as Consortium for the Barcode of Life (CBOL) that's international presence is dedicated to the development of DNA barcoding as a global standard for species identification. Like this international and somehow respected agency, Gates, and the elites behind all of this, desire to use nanotechnology to bring about synthetic changes to the natural body. Solum declares,

"It is not about the virus; it's about transforming everybody's body."

She goes on to explain the many variations of reactions people are experiencing due to the trial vaccines are a result of these artificial devices or synthetic cells, releasing different payloads of material in different parts of the body. An idea that is congruent with the ideas of various other credible sources. Like pathologists, epidemiologists, scientists, and other specialists, from other sources speak out about the artificially induced phagocytosis and manipulation of natural cellular DNA by the spike-protein antibodies produced in the experimental vaccines,

Solum describes the exact same process in her theory. All of this seems extra-terrestrial and at several points, I had felt overwhelmingly odd when watching these sorts of things formulate before my eyes into explanations for what could actually be occurring in reality.

Many of the COVID-19 regime's "fact-checkers" attempt to belittle and demean Solum herself and all of her claims. An intelligent person, however, knows how to follow a pattern. This COVID-19 regime deploys its fact-checkers to do the exact same thing to anyone and everyone who expresses a voice or opinion that may undermine its own credibility or mass fabrications. Like the story of the little boy who cries wolf…the COVID-19 regime or elites have cried wolf too many times to count and have even found themselves spun in a web of their own lies. Tread with caution if you are one who is choosing to side with them and their beliefs. Continue to do your own research and to think for yourself. Facts do not lie…people lie. For the first time, I am going to unpack that. Facts presented by people who have nothing to gain but your attention and the reassurance that by listening, you are then enabled to make sound and safe decisions and not be cornered or pressured into believing what is being said, are ten times more likely to be sourced in fact. Mass media represents "people lying," because they have something to gain, they have a track record full of manipulation, they instill hysteria, and they attack whenever the light is shined on them and their stories. There is an expression I had once heard and enjoyed while in biology lab at Clemson University,

"Look into the magnifying glass, and when you shine the light or stir the plate, you'll know which cells you are looking for because they will start to dance for you."

HOW A SINGLE VIRUS BROUGHT HUMANITY TO ITS KNEES

We the People and Freedom of Health

"You wouldn't abandon ship in a storm just because you couldn't control the winds."

— Thomas More, Utopia

With two defined sides, the world is in a war of information and pandemic. On one side, there are people who believe that the COVID-19 pandemic is exactly as the government, WHO, and mass media, say it is and more. These people also blindly embrace mass vaccination without contemplation or personal research. It is often the blind who fall into the trap holes set by sadistic and tyrannical authority. Birds of the sea, squalling over beachgoers waiting for tossed scraps, these are people of sloth and convenience. This group only receives the information that is shared from this front and all other views are either not considered at all or dubiously dismissed as conspiracy and falsity.

Across the battlefield, there are people who believe that the COVID-19 pandemic is less a biological threat and more a political operation. This groups believes what the government, WHO, and mass media, say, to be mass hysteria and hyperbole. These people also refuse mass vaccination with the COVID-19 experimental drugs because they conduct thorough research and make educated decisions about their health based upon the proven medical science. Owls in the night, observing and hunting in the darkness for what is being hidden from the light, these are people of action and opportunity. This group of people considers the opinions and information from all fronts and only accepts proven fact to be truth. It is often the sharp-eye and prudent who dodge and reveal the trap holes set by sadistic and tyrannical authorities.

It is unfortunate, that the people who are sightlessly conforming to what is being mass disseminated to them, are creating an enemy out of the people who are in opposition of this hysteria and attack on the basic human rights and civil liberties of the world population. To me, it does not matter how you feel about the

COVID-19 pandemic and experimental vaccines, so long as you are sourcing your information and basing your personal decision on your own observation and research. I am firm believer in what Thomas More writes,

"It is only natural, of course, that each man should think his own opinions best: the crow loves his fledgling, and the ape his cub."

Everyone is entitled to his or her own opinion and by holding a personal opinion, one is merely expressing a natural function of human consciousness. In principle, the passion behind the arguments made in this work comes from a strong desire to inform the uninformed and to encourage those who lack necessary initiative to research before they decide. Mass media is grossly benefitting by the throngs of people who are failing to practice this intellectual discernment. And they are not the only ones who are swimming in pecuniary pools of blood money. It takes a pound of physical courage to wield a sword on a battlefield, but only an ounce of moral courage to stand up for what you know to be ethically and morally wrong. Moral courage weighs far heavier than physical courage and this is the kind of bravery that it takes to become properly informed before making important decisions and having the ability to then stand behind those decisions. Between us people, there should be no war of information and pandemic. Between us people, there should be no racism and prejudice. Between us people, there should only be a unanimous respect for one another's differences in person and in views. We the people, hold the power in any nation. There is no need for a king or queen if there are no people to rule and there is no place for people where a king or queen can rule corruptly. In America and any republic nation actively practicing democracy, it will do a people great justice to be reminded of their government's roots:

"We the people of the United States, in order to form a more perfect union, establish justice, ensure domestic tranquility, provide for the common defense, promote the general welfare, and secure the blessings of liberty to ourselves and our posterity, do ordain and establish this constitution for the United States of America."

HOW A SINGLE VIRUS BROUGHT HUMANITY TO ITS KNEES

Belonging to such a republic entitles the people to a freedom of opinion during this difficult time. But to whom an information war must continue to be waged against, is the dishonest and corrupt elite agencies and individuals providing disinformation and half-truths to the world. If you are among the mentally blind, who willingly or carelessly, choose not to decide what to believe and what to do on their own record, you are enabling this enemy to the people and to the truth. Not only as a bias contender who has taken arms against such an ignorant approach of sloth by way of using the press and yielding the pen, but also as a fellow person, I urge you to start making decisions for yourself and begin to mine for your own information as opposed to only being filled with the white noise of mass media. To those who are only accepting the mass vaccination because they are afraid, uninformed, or are doing so only for sake of convenience, stop immediately and contemplate the sources provided herein and those gleaned during your own period of research. If you have already received the trial vaccines, learn this lesson to be better equipped for future scenarios. It is a person's freedom of health to choose whether to partake in a global experiment or to assume the potential risks of simply facing the possibility of contracting a virus someday. For these leaders and elites to be mandating, incentivizing, or pressuring, us people into making a direly important decision about our health and wellbeing, is a great misdeed and act of insidious tyranny. This is a battle to defend the people's freedom of health, press, speech, and decision. All of which are being challenged or stripped away by a common foe. We the people, not of nation, but of the humanity, need to unite against this enemy and danger to global public health. I implore of even those who have personally decided to believe the information that mass media has been pushing out to the world, to stand up and fight for the protection of human rights and civil freedoms of all of mankind. This greatly depressing situation has provided an equally optimistic opportunity to change how people are treated by authorities worldwide. Would you not like to see an end to police violence against African Americans and minority groups? How happy would it make you to help the people of a nation where leaders cause mass starvation and poverty, stand up and fight for proper provisions? These things are not possible when there are powerful and evil forces diabolically working against any such progress, which continue to be left unchallenged. Do not simply conform and accept the great mistreatment of the people during this crisis. So, what if you want to receive the vaccine; I do not! It is as much of a right for me to decide not to take it as it is for you to decide to. There is not enough evidence to support the safety or effectuality of these trial vaccines so by even restricting us people who wish to not be vaccinated and subjecting us to unmerited discrimination, is a direct attack to the constitution of **we the people of the world.** You are vaccinated, so why should you care or even bother to help the millions of people who do not desire to participate? Because as I have stated before, we are ultimately on the same side and so therefore, this abuse taken against a part of us will eventually lead to an abuse taken against all of us as a whole.

When viewed in whole, this work has primarily carried a negative connotation. Rightfully so, because the COVID-19 era is proving to be a historically depressing event. We discussed a myriad of different views and opinions and have explored evidence and research that contradicts what is being distributed via the mainstream. Instead of safeguarding the population against a virus, many of the governments around the world have capitalized on tragedy and used this time to increase their power over the people. Contrary to the lack of mainstream media coverage, in the United Kingdom alone, thousands upon thousands of Brits are storming the streets and opposing the lockdowns, mask mandates, and draconian measures, that have been in place for over one year. The government leaders are using the situation to manipulate and entice the people to do what they want. For example, the government is telling its people that if they take the vaccine, then they will have more freedoms; if they wear a mask, then they can go to the grocery store. One major problem with this abuse and yo-yoing is the fact that the overall elasticity between government control and people's freedoms grows lesser and lesser. Imagine a rubber band; the smaller it gets, the less elastic and tighter it becomes. With too much power, these elite agencies and leaders have continuously produced an onslaught of null and void reports and statistics of number of cases and deaths due to COVID-19. This was evidenced in the U.S. especially, where a myriad of physicians presented proof of a state mandated order instructing doctors to record as many cases and deaths as possible, as being COVID-19 related whether the virus was the actual cause or not. Some who oppose the necessity and claims of effectivity of mask mandates view the use of masks as a way to politically tag a person and therefore, create prejudice between those who are in support of mask mandates and those who are not. Grand divisions amongst the people are the greatest enablers to authoritative manipulation and tyranny. All politics aside, the evidence suggesting that there are sinister plans afoot aiming to depopulate or genetically change humanity, is worse than any attempts of authorities and leaders to abuse power and people. However, it is the proven susceptibility of these leaders and authorities to being influenced by these insidious agencies and individuals such as Bill Gates and his various subsidiaries, that poses the greatest threats against mankind and life as we know it. Studies and scientific research in things such as theragrippers, which are micronanobots that are injected into an area of mucosa lining and used to release doses of drugs into a subject, or Gate's 'Quantum Dot,' would enable these sadistic plans to be deployed against world populations. While juxtaposing his Utopia with realistic society, More writes,

"We did not ask if he had seen any monsters, for monsters have ceased to be news. There is never any shortage of horrible creatures who prey on human beings, snatch away their food, or devour whole populations; but examples of wise social planning are not so easy to find."

This is not a time for government leaders to be paying ear to individuals or agencies with this insidious nature. It is also not a time for leaders and authorities to be testing and depriving people of their freedoms and rights. Finally, it is not a time for leaders and world authorities to be permitting mass media to mass manipulate with disinformation and fallacious hyperbole. There has never been a time that requires the truth and transparency more than the COVID-19 era. Effective social planning with respect to people's rights and freedoms is needed more than ever before. As More confirms, there are no shortage of monsters in society that wish to do nothing more than to control, manipulate, or destroy humanity.

By ending any work of my own on anything but a note of hope and of positivity, I would be denying the frequency of my heart, mind, and soul. Let it be known, there is reason to hope and there is reason for hope. Humanity has endured many trials through terror and harnessed hope in the darkest hours. There is no greater evidence than this, that we will yet again prevail and overcome the COVID-19 pandemic and the mires of doubt and obstacles that have added to our great sufferings. In perhaps times of even greater darkness and despair, a young girl named Anne Frank shined this message,

"It's really a wonder that I haven't dropped all my ideals because they seem so absurd and impossible to carry out. Yet I keep them, because in spite of everything, I still believe that people are really good at heart."

Do your part and shine a message of hope to your neighbor, demand the truth from your superiors, and stand up against those who wish to bring us all into harm's way. With a united morality, we will become the social guillotine that is necessary to purge the world from these insidious agendas.

There is a legend about a small child who was once told by an old woman that an old and magical church lied beneath the sea. She specified that only those who truly tried would ever be able to hear the bells and that one day, if they continued to listen for the sound, they would finally see it. Very few ever heard the legend, fewer ever heard the bells ringing, and only the old woman and the child ever saw the old magical church. Listening for the truth and attuning your mind to interpret and receive only what are the facts in this COVID-19 drama, is like listening for the bells of a church that cannot be seen. Instead of the sound of the ocean waves crashing against the surf and masking the sound of magical bells, the incredible amount of misinformation coming from a myriad of sources, becomes the very muffler deafening the world's ears to the magic that only comes from focusing on the sounds of fact and truth. There are seven billion people living on our planet today. That means that there are seven billion individual universes, all possessing their own galaxies of thought and reason, their own planets of desires and belief, and their own stars of memories and mission. Never judge someone whom you do not understand and have never yet began to explore. The majority of people are choosing to ignore the bells of truth and fact ringing before them, but it is not one person's place to judge another person for their personal choice. It is, however, the duty of anyone who has chosen to listen to the bells of factuality, to translate fiction into fact and fear into forwardness. Let us work together to change our world into a place where the people hold the power and where the truth outvoices the lies.

"I must not fear. Fear is the mind-killer. Fear is the little-death that brings total obliteration. I will face my fear. I will permit it to pass over me and through me. And when it has gone past, I will turn the inner eye to see its path. Where the fear has gone there will be nothing. Only I will remain."

—Frank Herbert, *Dune*

About the Author

Joseph William Grieco was born in southern New Jersey and is the second oldest of four boys. In the middle of his high school career, his mother moved the family to South Carolina. It was here in the heart of the south where our author truly blossomed. Transcending the expected struggles often faced by young teens transitioning into a new school, he graduated top of his class. Since the first time he was able to wield a pen, he has been bringing stories to life on paper. In light of the COVID-19 pandemic, he was growing more and more distraught. Besides the draconian prison that the Italian government had enforced, there was an over abundance of misinformation and hysteria spreading like wildfire. He began to thirst for answers and this project was born. Like sheep, large populations of people were signing up to the amorphous agendas of mass media, WHO, and government leaders, without thinking for a second whether the facts added up. It is with a hope to enlighten these people, that he took on the onerous task of research and writing. The work that you are holding is the product, the literary blood, of a week of tirelessly researching and writing.

He is currently living in Naples Italy and is still actively serving his country and allied NATO forces. During the first COVID-19 lockdown, he also established the "Auxiluim" brand and began offering coaching in life, fitness and nutrition to people from all around the world. Grieco had also started up the "Auxiluim Ignited Podcast" show which he continues to host incredibly inspiring guests who with the hope to motivate as many people as possible to reach for their dreams and not to allow these negative circumstances to defeat them! The podcast can be found on Spotify. His other works consist of the *Cardinal Cure Series* trilogy: "The Memory: A journey of the heart and the mind", "The Dream: When Stars Fall", and "The Moment: Where it All Ends, It Begins".

Back in Florida, he has one son who is living with his mother and stepfather. Joseph has an insatiable passion for medicine and adventure, love, and culture. His many travels throughout the world have provided much of the inspiration he needed to finish these works. If there is one thing that he has learned from his almost three decades of life, it is that pain and hardship can be a portal to passion and progression.

Complete Bibliography

(I have tried my best to keep this list of references in chronological order in accordance with the flow of the work to make "source-checking" easier for the reader)

Zhou, Peng, and Zheng-Li Shi. "SARS-CoV-2 Spillover Events." *Science*, American Association for the Advancement of Science, 8 Jan. 2021, science.sciencemag.org/content/371/6525/120.

Shah, Ain Umaira Md, et al. "COVID-19 Outbreak in Malaysia: Actions Taken by the Malaysian Government." *International Journal of Infectious Diseases*, Elsevier, 2 June 2020, www.sciencedirect.com/science/article/pii/S1201971220304008.

Center for Devices and Radiological Health, FDA DICE. "Risk of False Results with the Curative SARS-Cov-2 Test for COVID-19." *U.S. Food and Drug Administration*, FDA, 4 Jan. 2021, www.fda.gov/medical-devices/safety-communications/risk-false-results-curative-sars-cov-2-test-covid-19-fda-safety-communication.

Offit, Paul. "Vaccine Development, Testing, and Regulation." *History of Vaccines*, 17 Jan. 2018, www.historyofvaccines.org/content/articles/vaccine-development-testing-and-regulation.

WHO. "Middle East Respiratory Syndrome Coronavirus (MERS-CoV)." *World Health Organization*, World Health Organization, 2021, www.who.int/health-topics/middle-east-respiratory-syndrome-coronavirus-mers#tab=tab_1.

Yam, Kimmy. "Anti-Asian Hate Crimes Increased by Nearly 150% in 2020, Mostly in N.Y. and L.A., New Report Says." *Google*, Google, 9 Mar. 2021, 21:37 CET, www.google.com/amp/s/www.nbcnews.com/news/amp/ncna1260264.

"COVID-19 Lockdowns." *Wikipedia*, Wikimedia Foundation, 28 Apr. 2021, en.m.wikipedia.org/wiki/COVID-19_lockdowns.

Hirsch, Lauren. "Travel Industry Could Lose $24 Billion as Coronavirus Cripples Tourism from Outside US." *Google*, Google, 11 Mar. 2020, 20:33 EDT, www.google.com/amp/s/www.cnbc.com/amp/2020/03/11/coronavirus-travel-industry-could-lose-24-billion-in-tourism-from-outside-us.html.

Lane, Rashon. "Mental Health, Substance Use, and Suicidal Ideation During the COVID-19 Pandemic - United States, June 24–30, 2020." *Centers for Disease Control and Prevention*, Centers for Disease Control and Prevention, 13 Aug. 2020, www.cdc.gov/mmwr/volumes/69/wr/mm6932a1.htm.

Wood, Donald. "COVID-19 Related Tourism Industry Losses in 2020 Topped $750 Billion." *Google*, Google, 8 Feb. 2021, www.google.com/amp/s/www.travelpulse.com/news/impacting-travel/covid-19-related-tourism-industry-losses-in-2020-topped-750-billion.amp.

Bartik, Alexander W., et al. "The Impact of COVID-19 on Small Business Outcomes and Expectations." *PNAS*, National Academy of Sciences, 28 July 2020, www.pnas.org/content/117/30/17656.

Erdbrink, Thomas, and Christina Anderson. "'Life Has to Go On': How Sweden Has Faced the Virus Without a Lockdown (Published 2020)." *Google*, Google, 8 July 2020, www.google.com/amp/s/www.nytimes.com/2020/04/28/world/europe/sweden-coronavirus-herd-immunity.amp.html.

Desk, Explained. "Explained: These Are the Countries That Have Not Imposed Lockdowns." *The Indian Express*, The Indian Express, 16 May 2020, 09:23:35, indianexpress.com/article/explained/explained-the-countries-that-have-not-imposed-lockdown-and-why-6389003/.

American Bar Association. "Two Centuries of Law Guide Legal Approach to Modern Pandemic." *American Bar Association*, Apr. 2020, www.americanbar.org/news/abanews/publications/youraba/2020/youraba-april-2020/law-guides-legal-approach-to-pandemic/.

BBC. "Earlier Coronavirus Lockdown 'Could Have Saved 36,000 Lives'." *Google*, Google, 22 May 2020, www.google.com/amp/s/www.bbc.com/news/world-us-canada-52757150.amp.

Sen. Marco Rubio December 31, 2020. "Dr. Fauci Lied About Coronavirus." *RealClearHealth*, 31 Dec. 2021, www.realclearhealth.com/2020/12/31/dr_fauci_lied_about_coronavirus_281464.html.

Alvarez, Felicia. *Bizjournals.com*, 15 Sept. 2020, 17:20 EDT, www.bizjournals.com/sacramento/news/2020/09/15/california-fitness-alliance-sues-newsom.html.

26, Rachel Cohrs Feb., et al. "Cuomo's Nursing Home Fiasco Shows the Ethical Perils of Policymaking." *STAT*, 25 Feb. 2021, www.statnews.com/2021/02/26/cuomos-nursing-home-fiasco-ethical-perils-pandemic-policymaking/.

Klein, Ian. "'It's Just Devastating': Mother Deals with Tragedy after Husband, Daughter Shot, Killed in Georgetown Co." *Google*, Google, 25 Aug. 2020, 13:51, www.google.com/amp/s/www.wmbfnews.com/2020/08/25/coroner-father-stepdaughter-fatally-shot-after-traffic-crash-dispute-georgetown-co/%3foutputType=amp.

Sawchuk, Stephen. "Education Week Stephen Sawchuk." *Education Weekly*, 2021, www.edweek.org/by/stephen-sawchuk.

Vanderwicken, Peter. "Why the News Is Not the Truth." *Google*, Google, 1995, www.google.com/amp/s/hbr.org/amp/1995/05/why-the-news-is-not-the-truth.

Lerch, Marika. "Human Rights: Fact Sheets on the European Union: European Parliament." *Fact Sheets on the European Union | European Parliament*, Sept. 2020, www.europarl.europa.eu/factsheets/en/sheet/165/human-rights.

Duignan, Brian. "Critical Race Theory." *Encyclopædia Britannica*, Encyclopædia Britannica, Inc., 2 Apr. 2021, www.britannica.com/topic/critical-race-theory.

Hartstone-Rose, Adam, et al. "The Three-Dimensional Morphological Effects of Captivity." *PLOS ONE*, Public Library of Science, 19 Nov. 2014, journals.plos.org/plosone/article?id=10.1371%2Fjournal.pone.0113437.

Kai KupferschmidtNov. 2, 2020, et al. "Europe Is Locking down a Second Time. But What Is Its Long-Term Plan?" *Science*, 2 Nov. 2020, www.sciencemag.org/news/2020/11/europe-locking-down-second-time-what-its-long-term-plan.

Blake, Aaron. "Analysis | Birx and Fauci Reject Fox News-Promoted Theory That Coronavirus Deaths Are Inflated." *Google*, Google, 9 Apr. 2020, 03:50 GMT+2, www.google.com/amp/s/www.washingtonpost.com/politics/2020/04/08/tucker-carlsons-brit-humes-faulty-theories-about-coronavirus-deaths-being-exaggerated/%3foutputType=amp.

Eurostat. "2020 Data on Weekly Deaths: a Peak in Late March-Early April." *2020 Data on Weekly Deaths: a Peak in Late March-Early April - Products Eurostat News - Eurostat*, 24 June 2020, ec.europa.eu/eurostat/web/products-eurostat-news/-/DDN-20200624-1.

Giuffrida, Angela, and Lorenzo Tondo. "'A Generation Has Died': Italian Province Struggles to Bury Its Coronavirus Dead." *Google*, Google, 19 Mar. 2020, www.google.com/amp/s/amp.theguardian.com/world/2020/mar/19/generation-has-died-italian-province-struggles-bury-coronavirus-dead.

United Nations - World Population Prospects<a href='https://www.macrotrends.net/countries/ITA/italy/death-rate'>Italy Death Rate 1950-2021</a>. www.macrotrends.net. Retrieved 2021-04-28.

Posted by: Team Tony. "COVID-19 Facts from the Frontline." *Tonyrobbins.com*, 7 May 2020, www.tonyrobbins.com/podcasts/covid-19-facts-from-the-frontline/.

Cassoobhoy, Arefa. "Herd Immunity: What Is It and Can It End The Coronavirus Pandemic?" *WebMD*, WebMD, 13 Dec. 2020, www.webmd.com/lung/what-is-herd-immunity.

Burke, Minnyvonne. "NBC News - Breaking News & Top Stories - Latest World, US & Local News." *NBCNews.com*, NBCUniversal News Group, 18 Nov. 2020, 11:41 CET, www.nbcnews.com/.

Executive Order. No. GA 34, 2021, p. 5.

PINHO, Ana Catarina. "First COVID-19 Vaccine Safety Update Published." *European Medicines Agency*, 29 Jan. 2021, www.ema.europa.eu/en/news/first-covid-19-vaccine-safety-update-published.

National Center for Immunization and Respiratory Diseases. "Vaccine Testing and Approval Process." *Centers for Disease Control and Prevention*, Centers for Disease Control and Prevention, 1 May 2014, www.cdc.gov/vaccines/basics/test-approve.html.

GLANVILLE, Daniel. "COVID-19 Vaccines: Development, Evaluation, Approval and Monitoring." *European Medicines Agency*, 12 Apr. 2021, www.ema.europa.eu/en/human-regulatory/overview/public-health-threats/coronavirus-disease-covid-19/treatments-vaccines/vaccines-covid-19/covid-19-vaccines-development-evaluation-approval-monitoring.

Liu, Mark. "Why the Johnson & Johnson Vaccine Is More Effective than You Think." *University of Rochester Medical Center Newsroom*, 13 Apr. 2021, www.urmc.rochester.edu/news/story/why-the-johnson-johnson-vaccine-is-more-effective-than-you-think.

HOW A SINGLE VIRUS BROUGHT HUMANITY TO ITS KNEES

Tribble, Sara Jane. "Pfizer's Vaccine Plant Has History of Recalls." *WebMD*, WebMD, 10 Mar. 2021, www.webmd.com/vaccines/covid-19-vaccine/news/20210310/pfizers-newest-vaccine-plant-has-persistent-mold-issues-history-of-recalls.

Pena, Luz. "Here's Why Some Are Experiencing Side Effects after 2nd Pfizer or Moderna Vaccine Shot." *Google*, Google, 19 Apr. 2021, www.google.com/amp/s/abc7news.com/amp/covid-19-vaccine-side-effects-pfizer-moderna-covid-19/10521642/.

Television, Daystar. *Vaccines*, 2020, vaccines.daystar.com/.

Craven, Julia. "Why We Don't Know What's Actually Going On With Periods and COVID Vaccines." *Google*, Google, 22 Apr. 2021, 12:17, www.google.com/amp/s/slate.com/technology/2021/04/covid-vaccines-periods-menstruation-side-effects.amp.

Kim, Tae Kyung, and James H Eberwine. "Mammalian Cell Transfection: the Present and the Future." *Analytical and Bioanalytical Chemistry*, Springer-Verlag, Aug. 2010, www.ncbi.nlm.nih.gov/pmc/articles/PMC2911531/.

9, Sherri Tenpennystated on February, et al. "PolitiFact - COVID-19 Vaccine Does Not Cause Death, Autoimmune Diseases." *@Politifact*, 9 Feb. 2021, www.politifact.com/factchecks/2021/mar/04/sherri-tenpenny/covid-19-vaccine-does-not-cause-death-autoimmune-d/.

GreatReject, "You Can Be Vaccinated with a PCR Test, Even without Knowing." *GreatReject*, 18 Feb. 2021, greatreject.org/vaccinated-via-pcr-test/.

Walter, Jan. "'T2K Neutrino Flux Prediction' on Publons." *Publons*, 2021, publons.com/publon/3705118/.

Frontnieuwswww.frontnieuws.comFRONTNIEUWS is tegen geweld. FRONTNIEUWS streeft naar een revolutie door de voorlichting van de massa. Wanneer de informatie beschikbaar is voor de mensen, et al. "Inmiddels 6.662 DODEN 299.066 GEWONDEN Gemeld: Europese Database Van Bijwerkingen Van COVID-19 'Vaccins'." *Frontnieuws*, 18 Apr. 2021, www.frontnieuws.com/inmiddels-6-662-doden-299-066-gewonden-gemeld-europese-database-van-bijwerkingen-van-covid-19-vaccins/.

GreatReject. "European Database: Meanwhile 6,662 DEAD 299,066 INJURED." *GreatReject*, 18 Apr. 2021, greatreject.org/corona-vaccine-adverse-death-injures/.

GreatReject. "Order Now: Your Personal Non COVID-Vaccinated Declaration." *GreatReject*, 27 Apr. 2021, greatreject.org/non-covid-vaccinated-declaration/.

Bernard, Dianne. *Three Decades before Coronavirus, Anthony Fauci Took Heat from AIDS Protesters*, THE WASHINGTON POST, 20 May 2020, www.google.com/amp/s/www.washingtonpost.com/history/2020/05/20/fauci-aids-nih-coronavirus/%3foutputType=amp.

Harmon, Kristin, and University of Wisconsin-Madison. *Bayh-Dole Act: Regulations Impacting Ownership of Patent Rights*, University of Wisconsin-Madison Research, 2021, research.wisc.edu/bayhdole/.

WwwAAASorg (Director). (2020, February 20). Bill Gates: How Gene Editing, AI Can Benefit World's Poorest [Video file]. In YouTube. Retrieved from https://m.youtube.com/watch?v=YNbOS4UBbDI

TEDtalksDirector (Director). (2010, February 20). Innovating to zero! | Bill Gates [Video file]. Retrieved April 26, 2021, from https://m.youtube.com/watch?v=JaF-fq2Zn7I

Fiore, K. (2021, April 22). Hospital to give covid vaccine bonus. Retrieved April 26, 2021, from https://www.medpagetoday.com/special-reports/exclusives/92216

Bossche, Geert Vanden. "Why Do Covid-19 Mass Vaccinaton Campaigns Promote Dominance of Selectve Immune Escape Varriants?" *Geert Vanden Bossche*, 31 Mar. 2021, www.geertvandenbossche.org/.

Chen, Yi. "Epidemiological Feature, Viral Shedding, and Antibody ..." *MedRXiv*, Yale, 20 Dec. 2020, www.medrxiv.org/content/medrxiv/early/2020/12/20/2020.12.18.20248447.full.pdf.

Gao, Leiqiong, et al. "The Dichotomous and Incomplete Adaptive Immunity in COVID-19 Patients with Different Disease Severity." *Nature News*, Nature Publishing Group, 8 Mar. 2021, www.nature.com/articles/s41392-021-00525-3.

Stamatatos, Leonidas, et al. "MRNA Vaccination Boosts Cross-Variant Neutralizing Antibodies Elicited by SARS-CoV-2 Infection." *Science*, American Association for the Advancement of Science, 25 Mar. 2021, science.sciencemag.org/content/early/2021/03/24/science.abg9175.

Bill & Melinda Gates Foundation. "Committed Grants." *Bill & Melinda Gates Foundation*, 19 Apr. 2021, www.gatesfoundation.org/about/committed-grants?q=Wuhan#jump-nav-anchor0.

Beaumont, Peter. "Tanzania's President Shrugs off Covid-19 Risk after Sending Fruit for 'Tests'." *THE GUARDIAN*, Global Development, 19 May 2020, www.google.com/amp/s/amp.theguardian.com/global-development/2020/may/19/tanzanias-president-shrugs-off-covid-19-risk-after-sending-fruit-for-tests.

Desk, Explained. "Explained: These Are the Countries That Have Not Imposed Lockdowns." *The Indian Express*, The Indian Express, 16 May 2020, 09:23:35, indianexpress.com/article/explained/explained-the-countries-that-have-not-imposed-lockdown-and-why-6389003/.

EngelBrecht, Torsten, and Konstantine Demeter. "COVID19 PCR Tests Are Scientifically Meaningless." *Bulgarian Pathology Association*, 1 July 2020, bpa-pathology.com/covid19-pcr-tests-are-scientifically-meaningless/.

Goloka. "Analysis of Test Sticks from Surface Testing in the Slovak Republic - Confirmation of Genocide." *Golokaproject*, Undisclosed School Laboratory in Bratislava, Slovakia, www.golokaproject.org/documentfiles/Analysis-of-test-sticks-from-surface-testing-in-the-Slovak-Republic.pdf.

Ghosh, Arijit, et al. "Gastrointestinal-Resident, Shape-Changing Microdevices Extend Drug Release in Vivo." *Science Advances*, American Association for the Advancement of Science, 1 Oct. 2020, advances.sciencemag.org/content/6/44/eabb4133.

"Consortium for the Barcode of Life." *Barcode of Wildlife Project: Consortium for the Barcode of Life*, www.barcodeofwildlife.org/cbol.html.

Creative BioLabs. "Custom MRNA Synthesis." *Custom MRNA Synthesis - Creative Biolabs*, 2021, www.creative-biolabs.com/gene-therapy/custom-mRNA-synthesis.htm?gclid=Cj0KCQjwsqmEBhDiARIsANV8H3ajYLwrUsmITtbCzHkiXH12zXFFDNv2sRCSBbfCIhQ4-ezunLkeeRsaAsrrEALw_wcB.

PUBLIC ENEMY #1: COVID-19

HOW A SINGLE VIRUS BROUGHT HUMANITY TO ITS KNEES